Contents

Chapter 6   Perming   111

Chapter 7   African Caribbean hair   123

Chapter 8   Shaving and face massage   153

Chapter 9   Indian head massage   169

Chapter 10   Improving your business   197

Chapter 11   Promotions and shows   223

Index   239

Advanced Hairdressing

3rd edition

A coursebook for Level 3

Stephanie Henderson-Brown
Catherine Avadis

Published in 2004 by:
Nelson Thornes Ltd
Delta Place
27 Bath Road
CHELTENHAM
GL53 7TH
United Kingdom

04 05 06 07 08 / 10 9 8 7 6 5 4 3 2 1

A catalogue record for this book is available from the British Library

ISBN 0 7487 9024 1

Cover photograph by Wolfgangmustain photography
Page make-up by IFA Design Ltd, Plymouth, Devon

Printed and bound in Croatia by Zrinski

Acknowledgments

The authors and publishers would like to thank the following for permission to reproduce material:

- BLM Health (p.16 bottom left)
- Cheynes: Jennifer Cheyne (p.103; plate 7, top left)
- Cheynes: Jack at Cheynes, Edinburgh (cover)
- Chubb Fire page (p.56)
- Clynol - hair by Michael Lewis, artistic consultant Headlines for Clynol; photographer Simon Bottomley; make-up by Carol Moreley; clothes by Rachel Fanconi (p.87, top)
- Clynol - hair by Susan McCafferty @ Krop & Co. Bathgate; photographer Simon Bottomley; make-up: Carol Moreley; clothes by Neil (for Rachel Fanconi) (plate 8, top right)
- Clynol - hair by Rusti Todd, Green Ginger, Newcastle upon Tyne; products by Clynol's Salon Exclusive Styling and Care collections; photographer Martin Evening; make-up by Carol Moreley; clothes by Rachel Fanconi (pp. 87, left; 89, bottom right; plate 8, style 2)
- Corel (NT) (pp.183-184)
- Corel 669 (NT) (p.125, top)
- Corel 730 (NT) (p.149, bottom)
- Darren Hau @ Headmasters; photography by Simon Coates; make-up by Mai Lee; products by L'Oreal Professionel (p.68)
- Denman (p.83, top)
- Francesca Gould (pp.169-196)
- George Paterson – La Belle Collection; hair by George Paterson; make-up by Suzie Kennett; products by Wella; photography by Malcolm Wilson (pp.130; 131; 142; 143, top)
- Goldwell (p.15, top)
- Hairtools (pp.39, bottom; 129)
- Haringtons (pp.68, top; 83, middle and bottom right)
- Headmasters artistic team. Photography by Simon Coates; make-up by Melanie Davey; stylist Zoe Lem; products by L'Oreal Professionel. (pp.68, bottom; 146; plate 1, styles 1 and 2)
- HEPR: Contemporary Hair. Hair by Alan Simpson and Karen Storr for Contemporary Hair in Guisborough, Cleveland; make-up by Carol Hayes; stylist Rachel Franconi; photography by Simon Bottomley; products by L'Oreal Professionel. (p.80; plate 7, styles 1 and 2; plate 8, top left)
- Instant Art/Signs (NT) (p.47)
- Institute of Trichology and the International Association of Trichologists (pp.15, middle; 16, bottom)
- Ishoka artistic team, Aberdeen; make-up and styling by Ishoka; photography by Jim Crone; products by Wella (p.226)
- Kerry Hayden (p.158)
- Laurence Bulaitis (p.128)
- Mark Glenn Hair Enhancement www.markglenn.com (p.88)
- Martin Sookias (pp.23; 73; 102; 164; 179-182; 185-196)
- Medusa Artistic Team at Medusa Hairdressing, Edinburgh, Scotland; photography by Jim Crone; make-up by Linda Wilson; stylist Angela Moffat; products by Wella (p.6)
- Nyxon (p.127)
- Photodisc 33 (NT) (p.149, top)
- Prestige Medical (p.39, top)
- Redken Laboratories Ltd. (p.15, bottom)
- Richard Ward © Richard Ward Hair & Beauty; photography by Joseph Oppedisano; make-up by Melanie Harris & Mark Hayles; clothes stylist Cannon; products by L'Oreal Professionel (pp.75, bottom; 80, bottom; plate 2, style 2)
- Saks Hair; Saks Art Team (UK); photography by Sheila Rock; make-up by Carol Brown (p.223, left)
- Sam Richardson photography (pp.69; 120)
- Sean Hanna Hair; colour by Fiona Connolly (p.87, left; 223, right; 224; plate 8, style 1)
- Sophie Butler Hairdressing; Sophie Butler, Sharon Payne and the Artistic Team of Sophie Butler Hairdressing, St Andrews, Scotland (p.70)
- Sorisa (p.39, middle)
- St John's Institute of Dermatology, London (pp.16, top; 17)
- Tom LeGoff/Digital Vision HU (NT) (pp.143, bottom; 151)
- Uxbridge College Training Salons (pp.76; 117; 125)
- WAHL (p.74)
- Wella (pp.75, top; 80, top; 84; 112; 197; 199)
- Welonda (p.154)

Every attempt has been made to contact copyright holders, and we apologise if any have been overlooked. Should copyright have been unwittingly infringed in this book, the owners should contact the publishers, who will make corrections at reprint.

The authors and publishers acknowledge HABIA as originators and copyright owners of the NVQ occupational standards for hairdressing.

Introduction

This book is designed as a guide for hairdressers undertaking the National Vocational Qualification (NVQ), or Scottish Vocational Qualification (SVQ) at Level 3 in either Ladies' or Men's Hairdressing. It is also intended for those wishing to enhance their technical hairdressing skills and expand their business knowledge. Advanced Hairdressing follows on from Basic Hairdressing by Stephanie Henderson. Written in an easy-to-follow style, it covers fashion styling and cutting for men and women, hair extensions, creative perming and colouring techniques, African Caribbean relaxing and thermal techniques, complex styling and locksing, shaving and face massage and Indian head massage. Also included is health and safety within the salon, client care and consultation, along with ways of making your salon financially successful, supporting customer service improvements and providing promotional activities.

Customers have increased expectations of all services and products available to them, and now demand both high-quality hairdressing and a complex variety of services to be on offer. This book covers **every aspect** of the new NVQ, including easy-to-follow guides from hair specialists Catherine Avadis on hair extensions and Yvonne Porteous on African Caribbean complex styling and locksing techniques. Specialist areas such as Indian head massage have been covered by material from Francesca Gould and men's shaving and face massage are also included to enable you to study, practise and then supply new services to your clients.

Hairdressing is a creative industry that allows individuals to progress through a variety of levels or stages. Within the industry, a wide range of opportunities exist, from stylist to salon manager or owner, from freelance or session work, to work in the theatre or television, and from technical work for product manufacturers to involvement in education and training. Whichever area you see as your goal, a thorough understanding of all aspects of the hairdressing profession is essential, and this book will be a valuable guide.

Chapter 1 Client care

The service given in hairdressing salons in the last few years has become as important, if not more important, to some clients and salons as the haircut itself. With clients becoming more demanding of professionalism and expertise from their hairdresser, and services and products becoming more specific, salons need to have in place certain policies with regard to the consultation process and giving clients advice on services in the salon and home maintenance.

This chapter covers the following NVQ level 3 units:
G9 Provide hairdressing consultation services
G6 Promote additional products or services to clients.

Client consultation

Client consultation means talking to your client and giving advice before starting work on their hair.

During this consultation you will also be examining your client's hair by brushing it through. In the same way that doctors diagnose their patients' illnesses, you will be able to diagnose any hair or scalp conditions and take the appropriate action. You will also be able to assess the client's requirements generally, and make recommendations for a hairstyle to suit their appearance and lifestyle.

Experienced hairdressers will be able to produce a perfect hairstyle for each individual client by considering:

- Face shape (oval, round, long or square)
- Approximate height (tall or short)
- Approximate size (thin or overweight)
- Approximate age (not everyone can take young styles)
- Skin colour
- Lifestyle (busy people want a hairstyle that is quick and easy to manage)
- Personality (quiet and shy or lively and outgoing)
- Occupation (some professions may have strict rules about hair length)
- Cost (make sure a price list is accessible)
- Medical history (some illnesses affect perming and tinting)
- Occasion (dinner dance, wedding)
- Time available (can the client spare the time for a long process such as perming?).

All this should be done **before** gowning up the client so that you can consider their clothes and lifestyle, and see their height and body shape more clearly.
Allow enough time to complete your consultation checklist.

REMEMBER

Clients may have no idea of what salon service they want. The consultation is your opportunity to make your recommendations and to build up a good relationship, which may lead to a return visit. Giving advice to clients about hairstyles, colours and products which are better suited to their look or lifestyle will promote the salon and yourself as an exceptional stylist.

REMEMBER

All consultations are done on dry hair before shampooing. You cannot always see the problems (e.g. dry ends) when the hair is wet.

HEALTH MATTERS
Standing all day long

Shoulders

Work with your shoulders relaxed. Exercise helps by contracting and relaxing the muscles. Try raising your shoulders up towards your ears and letting them drop. Do this six times in ten seconds, and repeat at least twice a day.

Gaining information

You must find out:

- The client's name
- The service (e.g. cut, perm, colour) required
- The chosen hairstyle (you may need to use a style book).

Don't forget that all salon records are confidential (those kept on a computer are covered by the Data Protection Act 1998) and must not be accessed without your supervisor's permission. This includes client records and staff records such as CVs, staff appraisals and disciplinary procedures.

Record keeping

Why bother to keep client records?

- A new stylist will be able to attend to a client when the normal stylist is away (off sick or on holiday).
- It is possible to check when the client last visited your salon for a colour or a perm (some salons send out reminder cards).
- Clients feel they are being professionally treated when they see you are checking their personal records.
- You are able to know exactly what perm lotion was used at which strength and what curler size was used on previous occasions (especially useful if the perm was too tight or too soft). Records of relaxers – the product, strength and development time – must also be recorded as they are particularly strong chemicals.
- You are able to know what make of colour or bleach was used on previous occasions, which colour was used, the peroxide strength and how long the hair took to process.
- Records of conditioning treatments will allow you to know how many were needed before the hair returned to good condition.
- You can keep details of any special conditions, such as any medication the client has been taking, or details of a resistant section of hair.
- You can deal with complaints more efficiently. For example, if a client complains that a perm has not lasted, but your records show that the perm used was a very soft one which was only intended to last six to eight weeks, you can remind the client of the details.
- You will have a record of the client's telephone number and address, which may be needed if an appointment has to be changed.

Records are generally kept for perming, hair colouring and bleaching, and for conditioning treatments.

Record cards

These are stored either in a filing box or in a filing cabinet, in alphabetical order according to the last name of the client. Cards must be filled in and replaced in alphabetical order after use. Some salons design their own record cards; others buy or use specially made cards.

Client name							Special notes	
Address								
							Homecare sales	
Daytime telephone no.								
Date	Stylist	Scalp condition	Hair condition	Technique	Products	Develop-ment time	Result	

Example of a record card

Computers

Many salons now use computers, not only for recording takings but also for keeping client records. To use a computer properly, you need training. All computers are operated by a program, which is known as the **software**. Salon computer software will be used to classify, store and retrieve information; the type of software used to do this is known as a **database**.

Once all client records are on the database, retrieving the information is quick and easy.

Contractual relationships

Some everyday things can be legally binding without you realising it, such as keeping appointments made. If quoted a price for a service they have received, the client must pay the full price. Many salons have consultation forms that ask the client to provide some personal information that may affect or prohibit the service to be provided. The client is legally bound to give you accurate and full information required. Because of this it is very important to have records of appointments made including giving an appointment card to the client. Quotes for services must be written down, receipts for goods sold and record cards showing the services given are essential if problems occur and legal proceedings are involved.

Client communications

REMEMBER

You must always be:
- Polite
- Tactful
- Honest
- Factual

during any consultation.

Verbal communication

Most hairdressers are excellent communicators because they develop good verbal skills through continued client contact. They build up relationships with clients based on quality of service and professional advice, by always promoting accurate information.

During the initial consultation you must ensure that you accurately establish your client's wishes, and that the client understands and agrees to what is finally decided. If you feel that the client is still unclear, then repeat a summary of the main information. Your communication skills are just as important when working with new clients as with regular clients, always promoting a professional salon image.

Listen to your client. Many clients never return to a salon because, although they may have been given a lovely new hairstyle, it was not the one they asked for!

Sample questions for clients
Here are some examples of questions to ask your clients:
- *'How often do you shampoo your hair?'*
- If the answer is 'every day', the client probably has greasy hair and scalp.
- *'How have you been lately?'*

  This gives the client a chance to tell you if they are taking any medication that may affect their hair condition.
- *'Do you have your hair permed or coloured?'*

  The client can then tell you about any chemicals they may have used on their hair.

Benefits of carrying out a good consultation
- Repeat business: a satisfied client will tell a few people about you, but an unhappy client will tell everyone.
- It will promote your salon's professional image.
- It will encourage clients to take up both existing services (such as perming and colouring) and new services that they may not have tried before, such as conditioning treatments combined with head and shoulder massages.

Consequences of not carrying out consultations correctly
The client may not only be dissatisfied with the service (for example, if her new style was difficult to keep because you had not suggested a light perm), but you could potentially damage the hair or scalp by failing to notice adverse hair or scalp conditions, such as cuts or abrasions on the scalp, before applying perm lotion. Salon business and potential promotion could be lost because of misinterpretation of the client's wishes. This could lead to mistrust, arguments and embarrassment.

Developing and responding to non-verbal clues

There are other ways of responding to your client as well as talking to them. People communicate non-verbally all the time, using both appearance and gestures.

Appearance

Hairdressing is all about creating images. Remember, not everyone wants a new hairstyle whenever they visit the salon. Many clients are quite happy for you to maintain the style they have, possibly with a few variations.

Personal hygiene

You will either be sitting or standing very close to your client during your consultation as well as when doing their hair, so remember that both bad breath (especially if you smoke and your client does not) and body odour can offend. Keep your breath fresh and remember that soap and water will remove stale sweat, while deodorants (which mask smells) and anti-perspirants (which reduce sweating) can help to prevent body odour.

Remember to keep your hands and fingernails clean and well presented. Nothing looks worse than chipped nail polish in the mirror as you are doing their hair! You are selling personal image and style to your clients. That means you have to lead the way.

REMEMBER
Clothing that is too loose may get tangled in equipment

Gestures

The obvious gestures that you should look for when selling products and services are:

- **Head nodding.** This means that a client is listening to what you are saying with agreement. A slow single nod means you should continue what you are saying; several quick nods means that the client wants to interrupt or make a comment of their own.
- **Eye contact.** By looking into someone's eyes you can soon see if they are feeling friendly or hostile towards you. When you are selling to clients, look them in the eye while speaking to them to gain their confidence.
- **Smiling.** Simply occasionally smiling at clients will automatically create good humour in the salon. It is very difficult not to smile back at someone who smiles at you!

TEST YOUR KNOWLEDGE

1. Describe how to communicate effectively with your clients.
2. Why is effective communication important?
3. What records are normally confidential in the salon?
4. Why should salon rules of confidentiality never be broken?
5. Describe four benefits to your salon of carrying out a good consultation.
6. Describe three consequences of not carrying out consultations correctly.

Developments in technology

Hairdressing is a fashion industry that is constantly changing. In order to be able to create the latest styles you must be able to use the most up-to-date tools and equipment and the most recently launched products.

To maintain your awareness of both current and emerging fashion trends and the latest developments in technology you should:

- Read trade publications such as *The Hairdressers' Journal, Your Salon* or *Esoterica*.
- Read general hair and beauty magazines such as *Vogue* or *Hair* which are available to the general public.

- Attend seminars and training courses, either 'in-house' at the salon or externally at a local college/private training centre/manufacturers' training school or hairdressing wholesalers.
- Attend trade events such as Salon at Excel, London.
- Attend hair and fashion shows such as the World Congress in London, the Alternative Hair Show and others in the UK and around the world.
- Watch television, not only for informative current programmes, but by watching some of the many training videos available.

Once you have this knowledge you should be able to:

- Offer the most up-to-date advice and the most complete range of services to clients.
- Know where to access new products/equipment needed in the future.
- Access new training courses to be able to keep up with the latest developments.

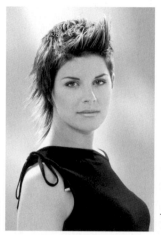 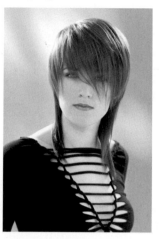

Recent styling innovations

medusa

medusa

TO DO

- *Describe how you could keep pace with recent developments in:*
  - *Cutting*
  - *Colouring*
  - *Perming*
  - *Conditioning treatments and massage*
  - *African Caribbean treatments*
  - *Long hair dressing*
  - *Photographic work*
  - *Motivating your staff*
  - *Health and safety*
  - *Interviewing techniques*
  - *Show work and promotions*

Examining the hair and scalp

Finding out what the client wants to have done to their hair and choosing a style is very important, but sometimes the client's hair and scalp condition limits the range of services you are able to offer them.

For instance, if the hair is untreated it means that no chemicals have been used on it, but if it has been chemically treated it will react differently to blow-drying and setting, perming, colouring and bleaching.

To undertake a hair and scalp analysis you need to section the hair in a 'hot cross bun' format, from ear to ear and from nape to front hairline. Then take each section about one inch deep horizontally across the two quarter sections at the back, repeating the inspection to the front (in the same way as stylists generally section off to apply tint to regrowth areas). This will allow you to observe both the scalp and the full length of the hair on different areas of the head.

A temporary colour (a coloured mousse or setting lotion) affects different parts of the hair compared with a permanent colour (a tint). You will need to recognise the different parts of the hair and learn how they are affected by various chemicals, and whether coloured hair can be permed, coloured or bleached in future.

HEALTH MATTERS

Standing all day long

Legs

Many hairdressers suffer from varicose veins, especially if they have had children. This is because they are not moving their legs when they are standing still and the blood does not circulate properly back to the heart. The result can be both swollen ankles and varicose veins (because the veins have become full of blue, deoxygenated blood).

If it is impossible to take a rest at work with your feet up, make sure that you do it at home by raising your feet on a stool or chair.

Exercise is the best way to prevent varicose veins. If you cannot walk or cycle to work, then try exercising in the evenings or on your day off. Walking is an excellent form of exercise.

Hair can be damaged by chemical treatments. It can also be damaged by handling – bad brushing, excessive blow-drying or tonging. Again, you will need to know what part of the hair is damaged and whether further services can be carried out.

As you are carrying out your consultation you can start to diagnose your client's hair condition. In order to understand why some people have shiny, manageable hair in good condition while others have very difficult hair, you need to know more about hair structure.

Hair structure

Each hair is made up of three layers – rather like a pencil.

- The outside layer, the **cuticle**, is thin and flat (like the paint on a pencil).
- The middle layer, the **cortex**, is the strong, main part of the hair (like the wood of the pencil).
- The central layer, the **medulla**, runs finely through the middle (like the lead in a pencil).

The cuticle

If you look carefully at the diagrams you will see that the cuticle is actually made up of **overlapping scales** (7–10 layers). These scales look like the tiles on a roof, with the edges all lying away from the scalp. They are translucent, like frosted glass, so that the hair colour (in the cortex) can be seen through them.

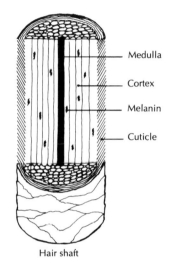

Longitudinal section through a hair

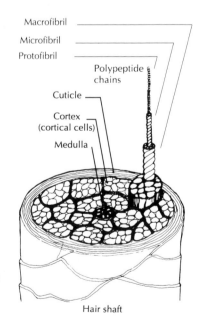

Cross-section through a hair

This outside layer of the hair shaft is very tough and holds the whole hair together, but it may be damaged by strong chemicals (such as perms or bleaches) or harsh treatments (such as over back-brushing).

If the cuticle scales have been damaged or broken and have opened up, and chemicals have been absorbed into the cortex, the hair surface will look and feel rough and dull like sandpaper. If the scales are undamaged and closed tight and flat then the hair will appear beautifully shiny like glass.

The cortex

The cortex is the main part of the hair, lying underneath the cuticle. Hairdressers need to understand the cortex because this is where all the changes take place when hair is blow-dried, set, permed, tinted or bleached.

It is made from many strands or fibres (the alpha-helix shape), which are twisted together like knitting wool. These can stretch, then return to their original length.

Hair is made of a protein called **keratin**, itself made up from amino acid units, which are found in long coiled chains called **polypeptide chains**. All the coils of polypeptide chains are held together by various links and bonds.

Look at the diagram below and find the **temporary bonds**. These are the **hydrogen bonds** and **salt links**. They break and rejoin whenever hair is blow dried, set, tonged or hot brushed into a different style. They are called temporary bonds because all of these processes can be easily reversed by dampening the hair and starting again.

There are also permanent bonds in the diagram: these are called **disulphide bonds**. Disulphide bonds are very strong and can be broken only by using a strong chemical on the hair such as permanent wave lotion.

The cortex also contains all the **colour pigments** in the hair. These pigments are called **melanin** (brown/black) and **pheomelanin** (yellow/red).

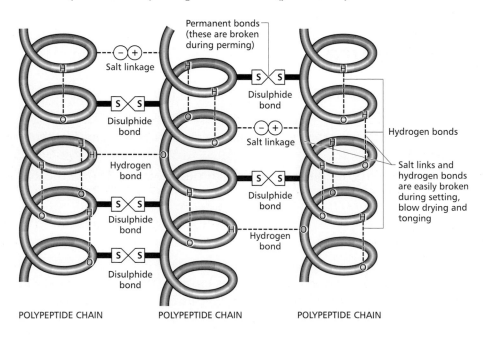

The structure of keratin

ADVANCED HAIRDRESSING

The medulla

The medulla does not have any real function. It is not always present in scalp hairs, particularly if the hair is fine.

Scalp (or skin) structure

There are two main types of hair on the human body. Fine **vellus hair** grows on the body; stronger **terminal hair** grows on the scalp and makes up eyebrows, eyelashes, beards and moustaches. A third type of hair, **lanugo hair**, is only found on human fetuses and is even finer than vellus hair. The scalp is stronger than the rest of the body skin (which is why we can put chemicals on scalp hair without causing too much damage) but its structure is otherwise similar to body skin.

Hair is made of the protein keratin, which is dead. There are no nerve endings inside hair and so it does not hurt when we cut through it, or when chemicals such as perm lotions or bleaches are put onto it.

However, we can feel someone pulling our hair because it is attached to the scalp by its root, sitting in a tiny pocket called the **hair follicle**. Nerve endings attached to the hair root tell us when our hair is being pulled and when a hair should stand on end. We all have occasional 'goose pimples', when our hair stands on end if we are very cold or frightened. The **arrector pili** muscle is attached to the hair root and contracts (or squeezes together) to pull the hair upright, creating the goose pimples.

The **sebaceous gland** is also attached to the hair follicle and produces **sebum**, the hair's natural oil or lubricant. The sebum flows around the hair root and outwards onto the scalp surface. If too much sebum is produced, the scalp and hair will be too greasy, but if too little sebum is produced the hair and scalp will be too dry.
The scalp (and skin) is divided into two layers:

- The outer layer – the **epidermis** – is the outer protective layer of skin. It is constantly shedding itself, losing dead skin cells. When this happens excessively on the scalp it is known as **dandruff**.
- The inner layer – the **dermis** – is the thickest and most important part of the skin. It is where the hair follicles, nerve endings, sebaceous glands, blood supply and sweat glands are found.

Hair could not grow without its own blood supply. The heart pumps blood containing food and oxygen (needed to make new keratin) through our arteries towards the skin surface. The arteries become **small blood capillaries** in the dermis, where they supply blood into the bottom of the hair root or follicle to feed the **dermal papilla**. The more blood flowing towards the hair papilla, the more the hair will grow. Therefore, when our skin is red and warm in the summer our hair (and nails) grow more quickly.

We can also regulate our body temperature through our skin because we have **sweat glands**. These produce **sweat**, which flows on to our skin through our pores, cooling us down as it evaporates.

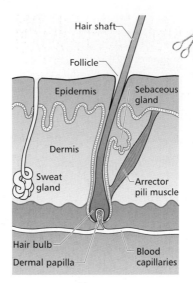

The structure of the skin

Ethnic structural hair types

There are three main racial differences in hair type:

● European (**Caucasian**) hair is oval in shape and usually waves easily.
● Asian (**Mongoloid**) hair is round in shape and usually straight.
● **African Caribbean** hair is kidney shaped and is usually very curly.

European and Asian hair (typically very straight hair found in people of Chinese and Japanese origin) react in much the same way to chemical treatments, but you will need to read Chapter 7, 'African Caribbean hair', for details of this hair structure and how it responds to relaxing treatments.

Hair growth and life cycle

Hair grows from the bottom of its root at the dermal papilla, where new cells are constantly being produced. These soft cells become hardened to form strong hair above the skin surface. The average rate of hair growth is 1.25 cm (0.5 in.) per month. This is what keeps hairdressers in business!

There are approximately 100,000 hairs growing on the average scalp, and there is a constant daily loss of 50–100 scalp hairs. We lose these hairs because every so often the hair follicle has a period of rest, and so the hair falls out.

The growing stage of the hair is called the **anagen** stage. When the hair starts to go into its resting state, it is said to be in the **catagen** stage. The resting stage is called the **telogen** stage.

Obviously not all hairs rest at the same time – or we would all be bald!

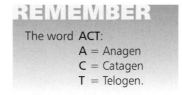

REMEMBER

The word **ACT**:
    A = Anagen
    C = Catagen
    T = Telogen.

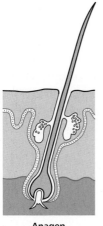 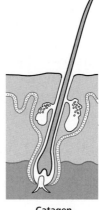 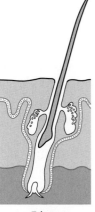 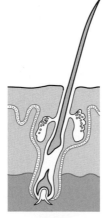

| **Anagen** Active growth 1–7 years (average 3 years) | **Catagen** Breakdown and change 2 weeks | **Telogen** Resting stage 3–4 months | **Anagen** Regrowth |

The hair growth cycle

The diagram above shows how the hair gradually stops growing and starts again.

Each hair grows for between 1.25 and 7 years before reaching a resting stage. This means that some clients' hair will grow to shoulder length:

1.25 years × 1.25 cm (0.5 in.) per month = 18.75 cm (7.5 in.)

but other clients' hair will grow down to their waist or longer:

7 years × 1.25 cm (0.5 in.) per month = 105 cm (42 in.)

So when a client complains that they cannot grow long hair you can explain to them that it is because their hair has a short life cycle.

TEST YOUR KNOWLEDGE

1   State a typical growth speed for hair.
2   Copy the hair growth life cycle diagram and try to label it without looking at this book.
3   Explain in your own words why hairdressers need to know about hair growth life cycles.

Hair thickness

This is known as hair texture, and it is determined by the thickness of each individual hair. Coarse, medium and fine hairs are large, medium and small in circumference.

TO DO

- *Pull out three hairs from your head: one from the front, the middle and the back.*
- *Ask several friends to do the same.*
- *Compare the thickness of each individual hair against a sheet of paper.*

REMEMBER
Some people have very fine hair, but plenty of it, while some people have very coarse hair but not very much of it.

Very fine hair

Average hair

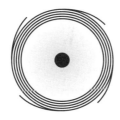

Very coarse hair

Hair thickness

Establishing hair condition

Like your skin, hair reflects your general health. Everyone should have a balanced diet and take regular exercise in order to keep their hair in good condition. Hair in good condition will shine and look great. Clients with a new haircut and this type of hair will also find that perms, colours and highlights take equally well.

LOCATION	GOOD CONDITION	POOR CONDITION
Surface condition	Cuticle scales lie flat and close together	Cuticle scales are raised and open, sometimes damaged. Surface is rough and dull, e.g. fragilitis crinium (split ends). Damaged cuticle. This is known as **porous** hair
Internal condition	Surface is smooth and shiny. The chemical links and bonds in keratin within the cortex are strong and elastic and contain natural moisture	The chemical links and bonds in keratin within the cortex have been broken by strong chemicals, e.g. perm lotion, hydrogen peroxide. This hair has lost strength, elasticity and moisture (through the open cuticle scales). It is known as **over-elastic** hair (stretchy hair)

However, hair that is damaged and dry may need special perm lotions or different types of colourants to improve its condition.

TEST YOUR KNOWLEDGE

1 List the indicators of hair in good condition.
2 List the indicators of hair in bad condition.

REMEMBER

● **Physical handling damage** is caused by bad brushing and combing (over back-combing) or excessive drying (hairdriers too hot, excessive tonging or hot brushing).
● **Weather damage** is caused by excessive exposure to the sun, sea and wind.
● **Chemical damage** is caused by excessive perming, bleaching (highlighting) and tinting.

Physical and handling damage

Here are some causes of physical and handling damage:

● **Bad brushing** – disentangling from the roots instead of the ends.
● **Bad combing** – over back-combing.
● **Over-drying** – the hairdrier too hot and held too close to the hair.
● Excessive use of **electrical appliances** – tongs and hot brushes.
● **Excessive tension** – especially from rubber bands.
● **Strong sunlight, sea and chlorinated water** – hair lightens/dries out.
● **Very windy conditions** – cause hair to tangle.

Chemical damage

You already know what chemically damaged hair looks like, but you need to know why the damage may have happened. For instance, a perm could look straight either because it was overprocessed (a straight frizz) or because it was underprocessed. The underprocessed perm could possibly be re-permed but the hair of an overprocessed perm would be sure to disintegrate and break off if further perming was attempted. The general reasons why hair may be chemically damaged are:

● Clients have used products from the chemist without any professional skill or knowledge.
● The hairdresser has not carried out a proper consultation or analysis.
● The hairdresser has misinterpreted the client's requirements.
● The hairdresser did not have enough practical skill, product or technical knowledge.
● The product was applied badly, left on too long (overprocessed), or not long enough (underprocessed).

Some specific reasons for chemical damage are:

● Perming – hair looks frizzy and may break off (the scalp may be sore or burned).
● Relaxing – curly hair has been permanently straightened and is starting to break off.
● Bleaching and highlighting – hair looks and feels 'straw-like' and the colour may be patchy.
● Tinting (tint applied on top of tint) – the hair feels very dry and the colour is patchy and uneven.
● Colour strippers – hair may be patchy in colour if strippers are not applied quickly and evenly.

REMEMBER

Always be tactful when dealing with incorrectly treated hair. Everyone makes the odd mistake, so be positive and helpful towards your client.

TO DO

● *Collect as many cuttings of hair in good and poor condition as you can find in your salon.*
● *Stick them down on paper and caption each with possible reasons for the condition.*

TEST YOUR KNOWLEDGE

State the effects of incorrect application of:

1   Bleaches

2   Tints

3   Perm lotion

4   Relaxer

5   Colour stripper

Abnormal hair and scalp conditions

These may be:

- **Non-infectious** – they cannot be spread from one client to another, for example alopecia (baldness).
- **Infectious** – they can be spread from one client to another, for example head lice.

Non-infectious hair and scalp conditions

Although a non-infectious or non-contagious disorder may be unsightly, it is not catching and can be treated safely in the salon.

Infectious hair and scalp conditions

Infectious or contagious disorders **must not be treated in the salon.**

Deal with the client sympathetically and tactfully. Explain that you have found a certain hair or scalp condition that means that you cannot continue with their hair service. You must then recommend them to seek medical advice from either a doctor or a trichologist (a specialist in hair and scalp disorders).

All equipment must be cleaned and sterilised after contact with an infectious condition (see Chapter 2).

REMEMBER

Do not name specific conditions when referring a client to a GP or trichologist because:

- The client may become anxious
- Litigation may possibly ensue
- Only experts can make an accurate diagnosis
- The hairdresser is relieved of the responsibility of diagnosis.

Non-infectious diseases

NAME	DESCRIPTION	CAUSE	TREATMENT	REFERRAL
Pityriasis capitis (dandruff)	Small, itchy, dry scales, white or grey coloured	Overactive production and shedding of epidermal cells Stress-related	Anti-dandruff shampoos Oil **conditioners** or conditioning creams applied to the scalp	Treat in the salon
Seborrhoea (greasiness)	Excessive oil on the scalp or skin	Overactive sebaceous gland	Shampoos for greasy hair. Spirit lotions	Treat in the salon
Eczema (sometimes called dermatitis)	Red, inflamed skin which can develop into splitting and weeping areas. It is often irritated, sore and painful	Either a physical irritation or an allergic reaction	Medical treatment	If the client is not receiving treatment refer them to their doctor

cont.

NAME	DESCRIPTION	CAUSE	TREATMENT	REFERRAL
Psoriasis (silver scaling patches)	Thick, raised, dry, silvery scales often found behind the ears	Overactive production and shedding of the epidermal cells. Possibly passed on in families, recurring in times of stress	Medical treatment. Coal tar shampoo	If the client is not currently receiving treatment refer them to their doctor
Alopecia areata (round bald patches)	Bald patches	Shock or stress. Hereditary (i.e. passed on in families)	Medical treatment. High frequency treatment	If the client is not currently receiving treatment refer them to their doctor
Male-pattern baldness (baldness, thinning hair)	Receding hairline, thinning hair. Baldness	Genetic or hereditary.	Medical treatment is being developed	
Cicatrical (scarring) alopecia	A permanent bald patch where the hair follicles have been destroyed	A scar from skin damage caused by chemicals, heat or a cut	None	
Sebaceous cyst (lump on scalp)	A lump either on top of or just underneath the scalp	Blockage of the sebaceous gland	Medical treatment	Refer to doctor
Fragilitis crinium (split ends)	Split, dry, roughened hair ends	Harsh physical or chemical damage	Cutting and reconditioning treatments	Treat in the salon
Damaged cuticle (tangled hair)	Cuticle scales roughened and damaged, dull hair	Harsh physical or chemical damage	Reconditioning treatments. Restructurants	Treat in the salon
Trichorrhexis nodosa (swollen, broken hair shaft)	Hair roughened and swollen along the hair shaft, sometimes broken off	Harsh use of chemicals, (e.g. perm rubbers fastened too tightly during perming). Physical damage (e.g. from elastic bands)	Restructurants. Recondition and cut hair where possible	
Monilethrix (beaded hair shaft)	Beaded hair (a very rare condition)	Uneven production of keratin in the follicle	Treat this hair very gently within the salon	
Keloids	Scar tissue with no hair follicle	Permanent damage to the skin	This area can be very sensitive, be gentle	
In-growing hair	Hair which has grown back into the skin	Looped hair which can be infected		Refer the client to a doctor and/or trichologist

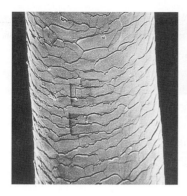

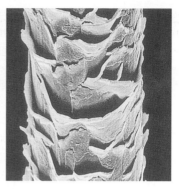

Smooth cuticles

Damaged cuticles

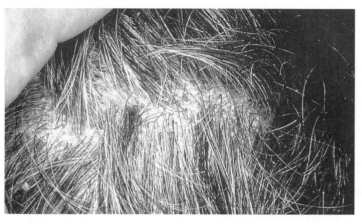

Psoriasis

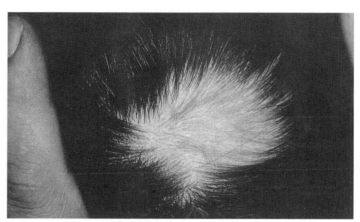

Alopecia areata

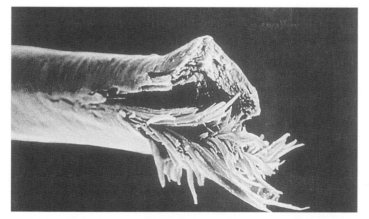

Fragilitus crinium

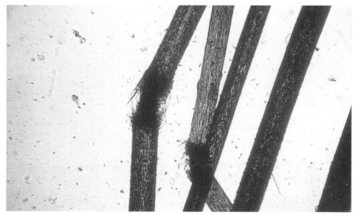

Trichorrhexis nodosa

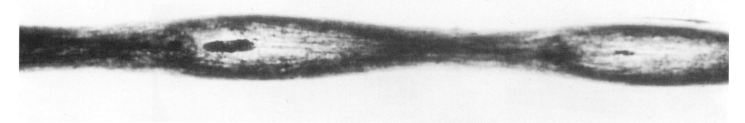

Monilethrix

Infectious diseases

If you suspect that your client has any of the following conditions, you must refer them to their doctor for treatment.

DISEASE	DESCRIPTION	CAUSE
Pediculosis capitis (headlice)	Highly infectious. Very common in children. Small, grey parasites with six legs, 2 mm ($\frac{1}{12}$ in) long, which bite the scalp and suck blood. The female insects lay eggs called 'nits', which are cemented to the hair	Infestation of headlice which lay eggs, producing more lice, living off human blood
Scabies	An itchy rash found in the folds of the the skin. Reddish spots and burrows (greyish lines) under the skin	A tiny mite which burrows through skin to lay its eggs
Tinea capitis (ringworm)	Highly infectious. Pink patches on the scalp develop into round, grey scaly areas with broken hairs	Fungus. Spread by direct contact (touching) or indirectly through brushes, combs or towels
Impetigo (oozing pustules)	Highly infectious. Blisters on the skin which 'weep' then dry to form a yellow crust	Bacteria entering through broken or cut skin
Sucosis barbae	Small yellow spots around the follicle. Irritation and inflammation of the skin	A bacterial infection of the hairy parts of the face
Herpes simplex (cold sore)	Fluid-filled blisters on and around the lips. The blisters irritate and swell	A viral skin infection
Folliculitis (small yellow pustules with hair in centre)	Small yellow pustules with hair in centre	Bacteria from scratching or contact with an infected person
Warts (small raised lumps)	Small flesh-coloured raised lumps of skin	Virus. Spread by direct contact. Only infectious when damaged

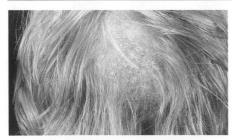

Tinea capitis (ringworm)

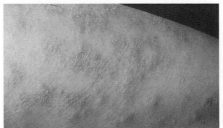

Scabies

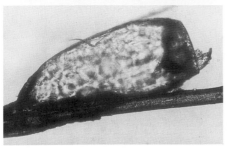

Pediculosis capitis (eggs or 'nits')

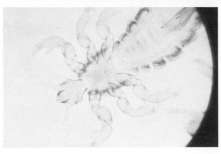

Pediculosis capitis

ADVANCED HAIRDRESSING

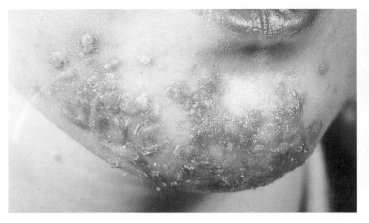

Impetigo

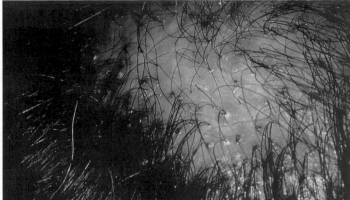

Folliculitis

TEST YOUR KNOWLEDGE

1   Without looking at this book, describe each infectious and non-infectious condition and its cause.
2   List which hair and scalp conditions can be treated safely in the salon.
3   Describe the treatments available for conditions that can be treated in the salon.
4   List the conditions that must be treated by a doctor.

Designing a hairstyle to suit your client

Have you ever wondered why two clients with exactly the same colour, texture and length of hair and the same hairstyle look quite different?

It is not only because of their height and build but also because of their head, face or neck shape. Clients must be advised according to these limitations.

Head shape

The shape of a person's head can be clearly seen when the hair is wet and combed flat against the scalp. For instance, if the head is flat on the crown you can compensate for this by leaving the hair longer in that area during cutting.

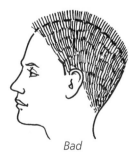
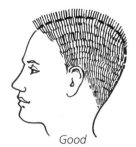

Bad   *Good*

Head shapes for a 'flat top' hairstyle

Head shapes can also be made to look quite different from the front just by altering the parting from side to centre. A side parting will make the head appear broader and wider, while a centre parting will make it look narrower and thinner.

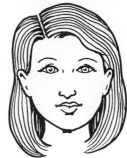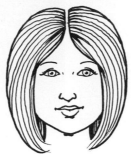

Side and centre parting

Face shapes

There are four main face shapes: oval, round, square and oblong (long).

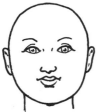

Oval

Oval
An oval face shape is ideal and suits any hairstyle.

Round
Round faces need height to reduce the width of the face. A straight centre parting will also help to reduce the width.

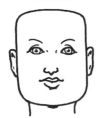

Round

Square
Square-shaped faces need round shapes with wisps of hair on the face to soften them and give the illusion of being oval.

Oblong
Long faces suit short, wider hairstyles dressed around the sides of the face. A low side parting will also make the face look wider.

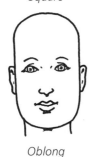

Square

TO DO

- *Comb all your hair away from your face when it is wet and try to decide on your own face shape.*
- *Make notes on your consultation sheets of different clients' face shapes.*

Oblong

Face shapes

Neck shapes

Long and thin necks are more noticeable with short hairstyles, and so need longer hair around them. Short necks can be made to look longer by an upswept or flicked style.

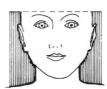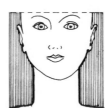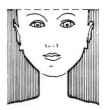

Neck shapes

Ear shapes and levels

Generally, large ears, or even large lobes, are highlighted by hair cut short or dressed away from the face. It is better to leave the hair longer over the ears.

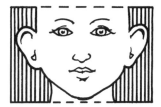 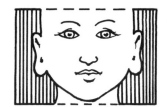 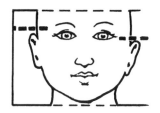

Ear shapes and levels

Some clients have ears that are uneven, so never balance a haircut by the level of the ears.

Nose shapes

A large nose will be more obvious from the side view when hair is drawn back from the face, whereas dressing the hair forward helps to minimise it.

Body build and height

One of the main reasons for consultation with the client before gowning up is so that you can briefly judge their body build and height.

Smaller clients can look overwhelmed by too much hair, or made to appear shorter from the back if their hair is too long.

On the other hand, large or overweight clients need a style with some volume and length to create a balance between their heads and their bodies. Short, flat hairstyles can highlight large bodies.

Age

A client's age is always an important consideration. Sometimes it is difficult to judge how old a person is, but generally softer styles with more movement are flattering for older people. Straight angular shapes are to be avoided.

Older clients also lose colour tone from their skin, so very few have naturally rosy cheeks; any redness is often caused by broken veins or cosmetic make-up. Dark or ashen colours can therefore be very ageing on older clients who, wishing to look younger, may want to return to the natural hair colour of their youth. Unfortunately this does not always suit them as they get older.

Client lifestyles

The client's lifestyle, occupation and personality are very important factors when choosing a hairstyle.

Lifestyle
The client could be a young working mother, who will not have much time to spend on her hair.

Occupation

Some occupations, for example the armed forces and catering professions, have strict rules about the length of hair.

Personality

A quiet, shy person may not be as daring with new styles as an outgoing extrovert. Clients are often worried about other people's reactions to a new hairstyle. A typical comment is: 'I'm not sure if my husband/wife will like it.'

Style books

Style books are very useful. They can be bought from hairdressing suppliers, or you can make your own. You can then adapt any of the ideas you have from the pictures to suit your individual clients.

TO DO

Make your own style book:
- *Buy a plastic folder with clear plastic inserts to hold cut-out pictures of different styles.*
- *Illustrate the front cover with your salon's name and logo and your name.*

You will need to include illustrations of up-to-date fashion trends, so try researching by:
- *Reading trade journals and magazines*
- *Reading hair and fashion magazines and books*
- *Watching television*
- *Going to hair and fashion shows, hair seminars and trade exhibitions.*

Organise the style book in sections, e.g. short styles, long styles, styles to show hair colours, styles to show different types of perms, styles for special occasions (e.g. parties or weddings), and to suit different face shapes.

TEST YOUR KNOWLEDGE

1 Describe how you can keep up to date with current fashion ideas and trends.
2 What type of reading information is available to help you keep up with changing fashions?

Hair growth patterns

Hair movement means the amount of curl or wave already in the hair, but **hair growth patterns** means the direction in which the hair falls.

This natural fall can best be seen on wet hair. If you comb your client's hair back from their face and gently push the head with the palm of the hand you can see the natural parting falling between the front hairline and the crown.

If you are cutting an all-one-length hairstyle such as a classic 'bob' then you must cut it to the natural parting. Otherwise, when the client tries to do their hair at home, the style could hang unevenly with long ends straying down.

There are several unusual hair growth patterns.

Double crown

If the hair is cut too short on the crown it is impossible for it to lie flat – the hair must be left longer.

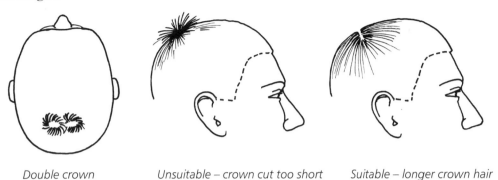

Double crown   *Unsuitable – crown cut too short*   *Suitable – longer crown hair*

Cowlick

This is found at the front hairline and makes straight fringes on fine hair difficult to cut. It is better to sweep the hair to one side.

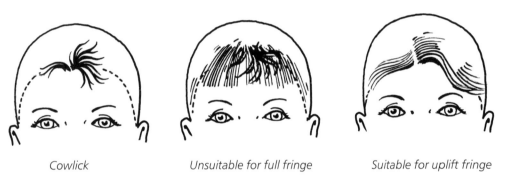

Cowlick   *Unsuitable for full fringe*   *Suitable for uplift fringe*

Nape whorl

This type of hair growth pattern makes straight hairlines difficult to achieve. It is better to cut the hair short into a 'V' shape or grow it longer so that the weight of the hair holds it down.

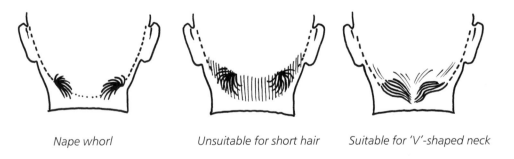

Nape whorl   *Unsuitable for short hair*   *Suitable for 'V'-shaped neck*

Widow's peak

This is where the hairline grows forward at the front to form a strong centre peak. It is difficult to create a full fringe because the hair tends to separate and lift.

It is better to style the hair back off the face or create a very heavy fringe so that the weight of the hair helps the fringe to lie flat.

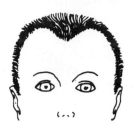

Widow's peak

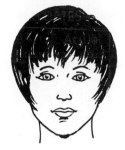

Suitable for heavy fringe

TEST YOUR KNOWLEDGE

1 List the different types of hair growth patterns.
2 Describe how a client's lifestyle can affect your choice of hairstyle.
3 Name the four main face shapes and describe a suitable hairstyle for each.
4 Describe how hairstyling can correct uneven head shapes.

Explaining hair treatments to clients

Once you have decided on the type of hairstyle to suggest to your client you should explain it in simple terms. If you go into hospital for an operation, the doctor will explain what is going to happen to you in clear non-technical language to make you feel much more confident. You should do the same with your clients. Don't forget that some clients can feel quite anxious about certain hair treatments such as perming or colouring and may need reassurance.

If you explain a conditioning treatment as a 'cationic, deep-acting chemical which is substantive to the hair, penetrating deep into the cuticle layers and helping to reduce the hair's ability to absorb atmospheric moisture', the client may become somewhat confused!

However, if you say, 'I'd like to apply some of our own deep-acting conditioner to your hair to help the dry, flyaway ends become shinier and more manageable', the client will understand more about the product and why you are using it.

REMEMBER

The client could potentially take legal action if hair and skin tests are not carried out and damage to the hair or scalp occurs.

TO DO

● Look up one method and procedure in this book for perming, colouring and bleaching. Write out a brief explanation of each in your own words.
● Practise explaining the procedures to friends before talking to your clients.

Hair and skin tests

Whenever you are unsure about how a treatment will turn out you should test the hair first. Hairdressers always use a professional colour chart when selecting a colour so that they do not make mistakes. Testing helps to make both you and the client feel more confident.

Porosity test

Porous hair can absorb liquids (water or chemicals) through the cuticle and into the cortex.

If the cuticle is closed, flat and undamaged, the hair will feel smooth. However, once the hair has been physically or chemically damaged then it becomes generally more porous or unevenly porous. This is why special perm lotions are used for tinted and highlighted hair, as normal-strength lotions could quickly overprocess or hair colour could become patchy.

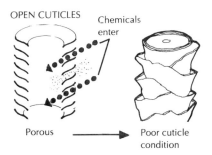
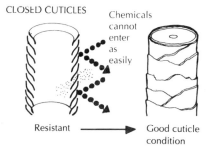

OPEN CUTICLES — Chemicals enter — Porous → Poor cuticle condition

CLOSED CUTICLES — Chemicals cannot enter as easily — Resistant → Good cuticle condition

Porous and resistant hair

Method
To carry out a porosity test, take a few strands of the dry hair and hold them firmly in one hand near the points or ends and slide your fingers along the hair towards the roots. The rougher the hair feels the more porous it is, and the more damaged are the cuticle scales.

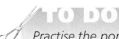

TO DO

Practise the porosity test on different types of hair.

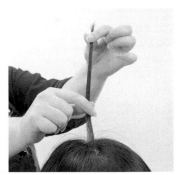

Porosity testing

Elasticity test

Well-conditioned hair is springy and bouncy; this means it has good elasticity. It can stretch up to one-third of its length when dry, half of its length when wet, and then return to its original length.

However, hair that has lost its elasticity because the internal chemical links and bonds in the cortex have been damaged may stretch up to two-thirds of its length or even break off.

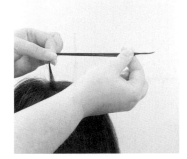

Elasticity testing

Method
To test hair for elasticity, take some dampened hair between your thumb and forefinger and gently pull. If it stretches more than half its length then it is over-elastic and may break off.

Incompatibility test

Some products that clients may have used on their hair may react badly with some of the chemicals that you intend to use – the hair may go green, steam or break off.

The most common products are **hair colour restorers**, such as Grecian 2000. They contain metallic salts such as lead acetate and the colour develops over a period of time. The hair often looks slightly greenish and feels harsh to the touch. The problem is that most clients do not admit to using them because they do not consider they are colouring their hair (they think they are restoring their natural hair colour).

In the salon a client with hair colour restorer on their hair must not have:

- a tint
- a bleach or highlights
- a perm (it is the perm neutraliser that reacts)

because all of these products contain hydrogen peroxide.

If you suspect a client has hair restorer on their hair, carry out an incompatibility test. Some temporary hair colours (colours that wash out of the hair), e.g. glitter sprays, also contain metallic salts and need to be removed.

Method

Mix 40 ml of 20 vol. (6%) hydrogen peroxide with 2 ml of ammonia (perm lotion will do) in a glass measuring container. Cut a few hair samples (use hair affected by metallic salts) from an unnoticeable area of the client's head and secure them with either cotton or sticky tape. Place the hair samples in the solution and keep them under observation. Results could take anything from one to 30 minutes to show.

REMEMBER

Always wear protective rubber gloves when you are using hairdressing chemicals.

If the hair has changed colour, if bubbles have formed in the solution or if the solution has become warm then there are definitely metallic salts on the hair.

Do not proceed with any hairdressing process that involves using hydrogen peroxide.

TO DO

- *Visit several chemist's shops and make your own list of all the products available that are similar to Grecian 2000 so that you can remember their names.*
- *Practise an incompatibility test when the opportunity arises.*

Colour test: taking a test cutting

In the same way that you would take a hair cutting for an incompatibility test from an unnoticeable part of the hair, you can easily test hair to see how it will take a hair colour.

Once the hair cutting is secured by cotton or sticky tape at the ends it can be tested with any of the following:

- Temporary colours – coloured setting lotions or coloured mousses.
- Semi-permanent colours – colour which lasts four to 12 washes.
- Permanent colours – tints that are mixed with hydrogen peroxide.
- Bleaches – used for highlights or general lightening.

Method

Mix a small amount of your intended product in a tint bowl and make sure that the test cutting is completely covered with it. Read the manufacturer's instructions to check the development time, but remember that the tints and bleaches will need longer than this to develop, because there is no warmth from the head to make them work. After the development time, rinse off the semi-permanent, tint or bleach products (temporary colours are left on) and dry the test cutting. With the client, examine it under natural light (near a window) and decide whether both of you are happy with the result.

Test cuttings are also useful to show whether the hair will take the colour evenly, especially if it is unevenly porous.

TO DO

- Take test cuttings from white, blonde, medium-brown and dark hair and try them out with samples of your salon products.
- Attach them to cards and record all the details.

Strand test

A strand test is taken while the following products are on the hair to check when the product has developed thoroughly:

- Semi-permanent colours
- Permanent colours (tints)
- Bleaches
- Colour strippers (colour reducers)
- Relaxers.

Method

Remove some of the product from a strand of hair with a piece of cotton wool or the back of a comb so that you can see whether it has developed properly, leaving the hair either the correct colour or the correct degree of straightness.

Development test curl

This test is taken when the perm lotion is on the hair during the development process. Once the curl is fully developed the hair is neutralised.

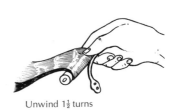

Unwind 1½ turns

'S' shape to size of curler

Taking a development test curl

Method

Undo the rubber fastener from one end of the curler. Unwind the curler 1½ turns, without letting the hair unravel completely. Hold the hair firmly, with both thumbs touching the curler.

- Using alkaline perm (P/W/) lotions: Push the hair towards the scalp, allowing it to relax into an 'S' shape. Do not pull the hair – remember it is in a very fragile state. When the size of the 'S' shape corresponds to the size of the curler, the processing can be stopped.
- Using acid P/W lotions: Push the hair towards the scalp and when it is developed it will separate into strands. This is called **stranding**.

TEST YOUR KNOWLEDGE

State how, when and why each of the following tests should be carried out:

1 Development test curl
2 Test cutting
3 Porosity test
4 Elasticity test
5 Incompatibility test
6 Strand test

Describe the consequences of *not* carrying out each test.

Skin tests

Many people suffer from allergic reactions to food or products (e.g. make-up). Hairdressing is no exception, and clients can become allergic to some hair colours. Permanent colours (which are tints mixed with hydrogen peroxide) and any quasi-permanent colours containing para dyes always need a skin test.

TO DO

- *Check the instructions on all the types of colours in your salon to see which ones need a skin test.*

Skin tests must be carried out before each application of the hair colour (usually between 24 and 48 hours before). If the client has a positive reaction (redness, blistering, itching, etc.) para dyes must not, under any circumstances, be used.

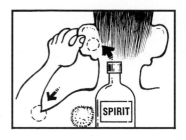

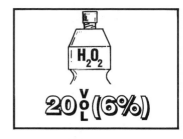

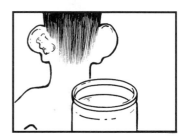

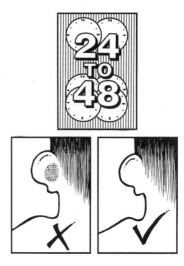

Skin test

Method

1 Clean a small, sensitive area of the skin (either behind the ear or in the crook of the elbow) with cotton wool and surgical spirit.
2 Mix a small amount of the colour to be used with equal parts of hydrogen peroxide, either 20 vol. (6%) or 30 vol. (9%).
3 Apply a small smear of the colour (about the size of a 20 pence piece) to the cleansed area. Allow to dry naturally.
4 Cover with collodian (New-Skin) and allow to dry.
5 Ask the client to leave the skin test for 24–48 hours, unless there is any irritation, in which case it should be washed off and calamine lotion applied to soothe the skin.
6 Note down on a record card which colour and which strength of peroxide you used, together with the client's name, address and the date.

Check the skin test when your client returns to the salon. A positive reaction (redness, soreness, itching or swelling) means that your client is allergic to the colour. A negative reaction (the skin appears quite normal when the colour is washed off) means that you can proceed with the colour.

TEST YOUR KNOWLEDGE

1 When and how should a skin test be done?
2 State the functions of skin tests in predicting reactions.
3 Describe the visible signs of a positive reaction to a skin test.
4 State the significance of a positive reaction.
5 State the significance of a negative reaction.
6 What could happen if a skin test was not carried out?

Consultation checklists

Once you have read this chapter and understood the variations in client's appearances and hair and scalp conditions you may find the checklists below helpful.

Checklist

Consultation and Diagnosis for All Salon Services

To be used for Unit/Element No _____ Formative/Summative

Date _____ Hairdresser's name _____ Client's name _____

❑   ❑   ❑   ❑

tick appropriate box

Client requirements

When was the client's hair last shampooed? _____

Scalp condition Possible disorder/disease _____ Dry/flaky/normal/oily

Hair texture Coarse/medium/fine   **Volume** Thick/medium/thin

Type Afro/Caucasian/Asian   **Movement** Straight/wavy/tight curly

Look Commercial/fantasy/avant-garde   **Condition** Normal/naturally dry/resistant

Previous chemical treatments P/W/relaxed/tint/highlights/lowlights

Hair growth patterns Nape whorl/widow's peak/cow lick/double crown

Testing procedures Elasticity/porosity/incompatibility/strand test/skin test

Present style Very long/long/medium/short/very short

Layered/graduated/one length/club cut/

razored/clippered/other _____

Client limitations _____

Any additional medical notes _____

Client lifestyle, personality, appearance _____

Client wishes _____

Suggested style _____

Shampoo/surface conditioner recommended _____

Conditioning

Time taken

Name of disorder _____   Product recommended _____

Massage movements _____   Equipment used _____

Cutting

Time taken [ ]

With/without fringe   With/without parting   Layered/graduated/one length

Club cut/thinned/razored/clippered/other _____

Styling

Thermal styling (African Caribbean Hair) Full head/partial head/tonging/pressing

Time taken [ ]

Tools used _____ Finger dry/natural dry/blow dry

Set description Conventional/alternative _____

Roller sizes _____   Pin curls _____

Styling products _____

Finishing products _____

Chemical treatments

Perming Virgin hair/tinted/bleached

Time taken [ ]

Pre-condition? Yes/No If yes, which product? _____

Winding method Root movement/uniform/non-uniform

Lotion type and strength _____

Processing time _____   With/without heat

Time taken [ ]

Neutraliser   Type _____ Method _____

Conditioning products _____

Relaxing

Time taken [ ]

Corrective/virgin/regrowth/remove curl/reduce degree of curl

Product _____

Method _____

Processing time _____

Colouring

Natural hair colour depth _____ % of white _____

Time taken [ ]

Temporary/semi-permanent/quasi-permanent/permanent tint bleaching/lightening

Full head/partial head/lighter/darker/highlight/lowlight

Product name and shade no _____ Peroxide strength _____

Method of application Conventional/alternative _____

Development time _____

Conditioning products _____

Client statement

Did the stylist discuss with you your requirements before any services began? _____

Was advice given for your hair and scalp care? _____

Did the stylist recommend products? _____

Will you consider following the recommendations? _____

Stylist signature _____

Client signature _____

Assessor signature _____

TEST YOUR KNOWLEDGE

When you are using a consultation checklist why must you always identify any limiting factors regarding:

- Your client
- The service being given
- The products you will be using.

Selling skills

A salon exists for one reason: to make money. Staff need to encourage clients to visit the salon and keep visiting regularly. The most successful salons are those with large, regular clienteles. There is no better advertisement than a satisfied client with a well-styled head of healthy-looking hair. A successful hairdresser must have:

- A regular clientele
- A good personality
- A strong sense of professionalism
- Good expertise
- The ability to sell themselves to their clients.

What to sell

Hairdressers not only sell:

- products – e.g. shampoos, conditioners, spray, mousse, gels, wax, etc. which enables the client to maintain the finished style
- equipment and accessories – e.g. combs, brushes, jewellery, hair ornaments, hairdriers, diffusers, tongs, etc.

but also advise about:

- the salon
- themselves (as stylists)
- salon services and treatments.

Therefore all staff must have a full knowledge of the services offered.

When describing the features and benefits of products and services you must be aware of the legalities involved. The Trade Descriptions Act 1968 states that you must not make false statements (lie about the products, features or benefits), mislead the client about services or products and you must not describe products falsely. The Sale of Goods Act 1994 says that the goods supplied you must be fit for their purpose (not out of date or broken), that they must be of merchantable quality (not about to fall apart or dangerous to use) and must fit their description.

If you are worried about chatting to your clients, try to ask questions that are open-ended, such as 'How long have you been coming to this salon?' or 'How do you manage your hair when you go on holiday?' These cannot be answered simply 'yes' or 'no', and help to get the conversation going.

Try to develop a **sense of tact**. Bad atmospheres can often be created by a slip of the tongue, e.g. 'My goodness, you do have bad dandruff!' Discretion is also important.

If one of your clients suffered from headlice, for instance, the worst thing you could do would be to tell other clients. Not only would these other clients worry that they might catch headlice, but gossip soon spreads and people might become wary of coming to your salon.

Try to increase your general knowledge by reading newspapers or by listening to news programmes on the radio. Once your confidence is established when dealing with clients, you can start to develop your selling skills.

REMEMBER

Never discuss religion, politics, sex or race with clients, as you can easily cause offence and find yourself in an argument.

TO DO

1 Open questions begin with 'How ...?', 'What ...', 'Which ...?' etc.
   Give some examples:
   'How _____ ?'
   'What _____ ?'
   'Which _____ ?'
   'Why _____ ?'
   'When _____ ?'

2 Closed questions result in a simple 'Yes' or 'No' answer.
   Give some examples:
   'Do _____ ?'
   'Have _____ ?'

Explaining various salon services

All the services that are available in your salon will be displayed on the price list. Clients will often ask about the benefits of different services. Here are some explanations you might give:

● 'Our reconditioning treatments work particularly well because we give a special massage to help them to penetrate into the hair.'

● 'We give two types of permanent waves. One is for a firm curl, the other is an acid perm which is gentler on the hair and will not dry it out.'

Here is a fuller description of a client discussion.

Discovering client needs
Stylist: 'Your hair has some pretty lightness at the very ends. Is that from your holiday last summer?'
Client: 'Yes, the sun lightened it, but it has nearly grown out now.'
Stylist: 'We could always place some natural-looking highlights through your hair to keep it going until next summer.'

Describing features of service
Client: 'Oh yes, how is that done?'
Stylist: 'By using either cap highlights or foil. The cap method is quicker and less expensive, but the foil gives more highlights exactly where you want them, and you can vary the colour.'
Client: 'What sort of colour would you suggest?'

Looking for buying signals
Stylist (*uses shade cards*): 'These light beige blonde tones exactly match the ends of your hair and would look very natural.'
Client: 'How long do they last?'

Describing benefits to client

Stylist: 'They will grow out gradually, and they give your hair a lot more body, which would help your fine hair to keep its style longer.'

Client: 'How much would they cost?'

Close sale

Stylist: 'They are normally £65.00 but we have a special offer of £55.00 if you can make a Monday or Tuesday appointment.'

Client: 'Yes, thank you, I'll make an appointment for next week.'

You can also use style books and product leaflets, rather than just words, to show the client what you mean. Clients will naturally want to know the cost of the service, so make sure you work it out correctly.

It is also important to explain to the client the length of time that different services will take. A short cut and blow-dry with little hair removed may take only 30–45 minutes, whereas a re-style, cut and blow-dry for a client with long hair which needs to be cut short may take well over an hour.

Retailing in the salon

All hairdressers have an excellent opportunity for selling products in the salon, in that they know what to use and how to use it. Once you have tried your particular salon mousse, for instance, you will understand its benefits (firm hold, non-sticky, gives lift, etc.) and find it easy to explain these benefits to your clients.

You can show the products to clients by the display at the reception area, but allowing clients to handle products also helps to sell them. If you allow the client to touch, feel or smell the product – especially when you are using it on their hair – you will always gain their interest.

Understanding your market

You will be selling hairdressing services and hairdressing products to many different types of client, each having different characteristics – long face, round face, high hairline, etc. This makes it important for you to recommend the correct product, service and hairstyle for each one.

Here is an example of how to sell a product.

Describe client needs

Stylist: 'Your hair is still a little dry at the ends; would you like me to use our new conditioner today, at no extra charge?'

Client: 'Yes please. What is this one?'

Describe product

Stylist: 'Well, it's one that you actually leave in the hair and don't rinse out. So it does save time.'

Client: 'Won't it leave my hair feeling sticky?'

Stylist: 'Not at all. Try a little on your hands. You can rub it into your skin and see it disappear. It works like that on your hair.'

Client (tries the product on her hands): 'Yes, my hands do feel soft and smooth.'

Describe features

Stylist: 'You can use it every time you shampoo your hair and also use it as a hand cream.'
Client: 'How much do I need to use?'

Describe how to use it

Stylist: 'Just squeeze out an amount the size of a small coin, rub the palms of your hands together and smooth the conditioner into the ends of your hair.'
Client: 'Can I buy it at reception?'

Close sale

Stylist: 'Yes, the prices of all the sizes are clearly marked. Remember you get a hair conditioner and a hand cream for the same price!'

Once you have gained some product knowledge, you will find the best way to talk about it is in this order:

1 Describe the product – what it is (e.g. shampoo, hairspray).
2 Describe how it works – what it does (e.g. especially benefits permed hair or hair that is washed frequently, or prevents salon colours from fading).
3 Describe how to use it – e.g. hold the hairspray 30 cm away from your hair, or shake the can immediately before use.

Use your common sense when selling services and products. For example, a young working mother with no time to spare would be more likely to buy a combined shampoo and conditioner or a 'wash 'n' wear' perm than a senior citizen with more time on her hands.

REMEMBER

● Whilst you are selling, use the client's name (it's the sweetest sound they know!)
● Learn to recognise non-verbal clues:
Dilated pupils
        = 'I approve'
Ear rubbing
        = 'I've had enough'

TO DO

● *Practise looking in the mirror and keeping eye contact with your client whilst selling to them.*

TO DO

Here are some examples of client types:

Young and fashionable	Senior citizens	European
Professional business people	Children	African-Caribbean
Students	Uniformed professionals	Asian
Young mothers	(e.g. nurses and police officers)	Oriental

● *Make a short list of the products and the services that your salon has to offer to suit some of the above client types. For example:*

Client type	Product
Young and fashionable	Firm-hold mousse, short clippered styles
Senior citizens	Regular use of hair spray, firm, curly perms

● *Make a list of the best types of tools and equipment your clients should buy to use at home and the correct methods of using them, e.g. brushes, combs, hairdriers and other electrical equipment.*

● *Re-read the section on designing a hairstyle to suit your client and make notes on which styles suit different client characteristics, e.g. round face, long neck, etc.*

Selling: the three stages

1 **Finding out the client's needs**. This means identifying any previous treatments or problems. You will have learned to do this tactfully during the consultation process. Examples might include fine, lank hair, itchy scaly scalp, dry, split ends, etc.
2 **Giving the client advice**. This means asking any relevant questions that will lead you to suggest a particular service or product. Here are some examples:
   ● Fine, lank hair – 'Have you ever thought about having a soft body perm which just gives volume and bounce?'

REMEMBER

Gain as much knowledge as you possibly can. Only when you are confident with the products you are selling can you be an enthusiastic and effective salesperson.

- Itchy, dry scalp – 'Do you find your itchy scalp becomes worse with certain shampoos?' ('We have one which is especially soothing,' etc.)
- Dry, split ends – 'How often do you have your hair trimmed? We recommend cutting every six weeks to reduce split ends.'

3 **Gaining agreement with the client**. This is achieved by either receiving an immediate response or giving them time to think about it. For example, 'Would you like a perm on your hair now?' or 'My hair has been easy to manage with this perm. I'm sure that yours would be too.'

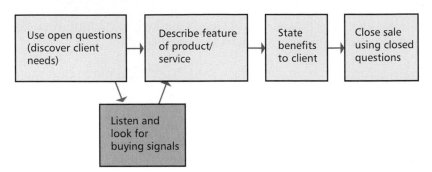

Finally, don't forget to record any sales or client services on your record card for next time.

Bad selling

If you were wondering where you went wrong, here are some common faults:
- Doing all the talking
- Knowing nothing about the product
- Interrupting – but not letting the clients interrupt you, thereby losing an opportunity for giving extra information
- Not listening, not 'hearing' unspoken thoughts, arguing
- Hard selling – working to a script, insisting the client buys the product
- Threatening – 'You won't get it cheaper anywhere else'
- 'Knocking the opposition', i.e. criticising other salons
- Manipulating – 'Oh dear, you'll make me miss my sales target'
- Treating 'No thanks' as a personal rejection
- Blinding clients with science
- Staying mainly silent, waiting for an order.

Client feedback

Client feedback should always be encouraged. It will help to improve your service and win repeat business.
It may be done in several ways:
- By using open-ended questions to obtain feedback from both your own clients and from the clients of your colleagues.
- By using client questionnaires (see Chapter 10, page 211).
- By having a suggestion box or a client comment box.

TO DO
- *Read Chapter 10, page 200, on problems that can arise in the salon. Describe how you would cope with a client waiting for an appointment.*

Whichever method you use, the feedback must be reported and passed on, so that it can be used constructively in the future.

Positive and negative feedback

Hopefully, most client feedback will be positive, but when negative feedback occurs, it must be dealt with in a professional manner. If a client approaches you with a complaint:

- Pleasantly and politely ask the client to sit with you in a quiet area of the salon so that you can discuss it in private.
- Talk through the problem together to diagnose the fault. When the complaint has been explained, repeat it back and confirm with the client that you have heard it correctly.
- Don't argue with the client – they will become more angry and create a disturbance in the salon. Stay calm, polite and understanding, never show your emotions. Try not to take it personally.
- Diagnose the fault and suggest corrective action.
- If the client agrees with your suggestions, then carry out the correction there and then, or agree a convenient return appointment.
- Always record the complaint and the action taken, and thank the client for bringing the problem to your attention.

TO DO

- *Ask a friend to pretend to be a difficult client with a just complaint about their hair. Ask another hairdresser to watch and comment on how you deal with the situation.*

Body language
Always take a deep breath and put on your most sympathetic face when faced with an angry client.

- Don't fold your arms – it looks too defensive.
- Don't lean too far forward – it may look aggressive.
- Don't make body contact – and keep a reasonable physical distance from the client.
- Don't clench your teeth, or tense your muscles – it may look as if you are trying to control your temper.
- Look interested and don't interrupt!

Ethics

Ethics is a code of behaviour considered to be moral and correct. An employee should:

- Set a good example of good conduct and behaviour in the salon
- Provide a friendly and courteous service to all clients
- Treat all clients honestly and fairly
- Provide friendly and courteous assistance to colleagues
- Practise high standards of hygiene at all times
- Show respect for feelings and rights of others
- Fulfil their obligations by keeping their word

TO DO

- *Draw up a 'Lines of Communication' chart for your salon, stating each person's name, roles and responsibilities.*
- *Describe how your salon deals with client feedback. For example, is it through staff meetings, reports from the manager or open discussion?*

REMEMBER

Your salon will be covered by insurance because of the Employers Liability (Compulsory Insurance) Act 1969.
This requires employers to take out insurance on themselves and their employees for accidental damage to themselves and to clients.

- Obey all provisions of government and law
- Be loyal to their employer.

Serious complaints

If the client's hair is breaking off or they have a sore, inflamed scalp and you have not taken the necessary precautions, then:
- Never admit liability
- Consult with a senior member of staff or the manager.

The senior member of staff or the manager must then:
- Notify the salon's insurers immediately that there is the possibility of a claim arising
- Pass on all correspondence, unanswered, to the insurers.

If the worst comes to the worst and the situation is not resolved to the client's satisfaction, then the next call could be from the client's solicitor, or from the news desk of a tabloid newspaper.

Always pass media calls to the manager or owner.

Remember that client record cards and completed consultation sheets which include lifestyle questions and medical treatments may be a good defence in a court of law.

Prevention is better than cure! If your professional opinion is that you should not do the client's hair, then suggest something like 'Another hairdresser may well do your hair, but I'd like you to be a regular client and I'd like you to leave our salon feeling happy, so please be guided by my experience.'

TEST YOUR KNOWLEDGE

1 Describe three different ways that you could obtain feedback from your clients on your salon's services.

2 Describe your initial response if a client approaches you with a complaint.

3 In the event of a serious complaint, what is the next step in the complaints procedure?

4 Why is it important to understand your salon's lines of communication when dealing with negative feedback?

Chapter 2 Health and safety

Issues of health and safety in the workplace affect everyone working in or visiting the salon. The responsibility lies with the workers in the salon to know and understand certain legislation regarding their day-to-day activities. General behaviour in the salon must not cause a danger to anyone else and hazards should be identified and dealt with immediately. This chapter covers the potential hazards and risks often found in the salon and how to deal with them.

This chapter covers the following NVQ level 3 unit:
G1 Ensure your own actions reduce risks to health and safety.

Working practices

Hairdressers must always work:

- **Cleanly**. Both your client's health and your own health are at risk. Tools and equipment must be clean and properly sterilised. There are many diseases that you and your client could catch from dirty equipment – such as headlice, impetigo and ringworm.
- **Safely**. Careless work could lead to hair loss, hair breakage, damage to the client's skin or eyes, or ruined clothes.

Did you know that legally you (the employee) must take care of not only your own health and safety, but also that of anyone else who may be affected by your work?

This means that both you and your staff should:

- Know where the emergency exits are in case of fire, flood, bomb alert or gas leaks
- Know how to telephone for the emergency services (e.g. the fire brigade or ambulance service)
- Know which chemicals used in the salon are dangerous and how to use them safely
- Know how to use electrical equipment safely
- Have some knowledge of emergency first aid
- Work with an awareness of security procedures
- Know how to store, use and dispose of stock, both for salon and retail use
- Know how to deal with suspicious persons and packages.

This applies to:

- Staff and clients, and their possessions
- The salon premises, fixtures and fittings.

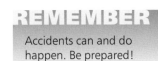

REMEMBER
Accidents can and do happen. Be prepared!

Salon hygiene

In order to prevent the spread of infection:

- Each hairdresser should have at least two sets of tools, one in use and the other being sterilised or disinfected ready for the next client.
- Clean towels and gowns should be given to each client. Towels should be washed and dried after use (not just dried).
- Hair should be swept up after every haircut and placed in a covered container.
- All work surfaces must be regularly cleaned with hot water and detergent. Surfaces should be made of materials that are free of cracks and are easy to keep clean.
- Clients with any infectious conditions (e.g. headlice, ringworm or impetigo) should not be treated in the salon but tactfully referred to a doctor. If work begins before the problem is noticed, then the service should be completed as quickly as possible. Contaminated hair (e.g. hair containing nits or headlice) should be swept up immediately and preferably burnt; failing this, it should be placed in a sealed container. Hairdressing equipment and clothing that has been in contact with the client must be sterilised or disinfected.
- Care should be taken when using tools which may cut or pierce the skin or in areas with open, bleeding or weeping wounds or cuts because of the risk of AIDS and Hepatitis B (see below). Disposable razor blades must be safely disposed of by placing in a secure container, such as a wide-mouthed screw-topped bottle or commercial sharps container, before being placed in the bin.

AIDS (acquired immunodeficiency syndrome)

This is caused by a virus that attacks the natural defence system of the body, preventing it from fighting disease or infection. It is transmitted by blood or tissue fluid from an infected person entering a break in the skin of a healthy person, and can be fatal.

Hepatitis B

This is a virus that attacks the liver. Hepatitis is a very serious disease that can kill. It is transmitted by infected blood or tissue fluid coming into contact with the body fluids of an uninfected person, usually through a cut. Therefore, combs, brushes, etc., should not be used on broken skin affected with boils or skin rashes (such as impetigo) unless they can be sterilised immediately afterwards. If skin is accidentally cut with scissors, clippers or razors, these must immediately be cleaned and sterilised.

Sterilisation and disinfection

All tools such as brushes, combs and hair rollers must be thoroughly cleaned with hot soapy water to remove loose hairs, dust and dirt. Scissors and razors can be cleaned with alcohol. This must be done before sterilisation or disinfection.

Sterilisation

This means the killing of all organisms, whether:

- Fungi, e.g. ringworm
- Bacteria, e.g. impetigo
- Parasites, e.g. headlice.

Autoclaves

These are highly recommended, as they are the most efficient way of sterilising metal tools, combs and plastics (check beforehand that tools can withstand the heat). Autoclaves sterilise by the creation of steam heat (121°C) and pressure. They take about 20 minutes to work.

Boiling in water

Towels and gowns should be washed in a hot-wash cycle, where the water should reach 95°C.

Ultraviolet radiation cabinet

These are used in many salons, but all the tools must be perfectly clean before being placed in this cabinet.

During the process, tools must be turned over frequently to expose all surfaces to the ultraviolet rays which come from a mercury vapour lamp at the top of the cabinet. Each side of the tools should be exposed to the ultraviolet rays for 20–30 minutes.

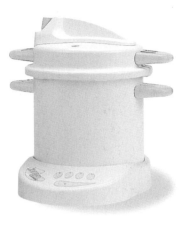

An autoclave

REMEMBER

If tools are accidentally dropped on the floor, they must be cleaned, dried and sterilised before being used again.
Broken tools must not be used because they can be a source of infection.

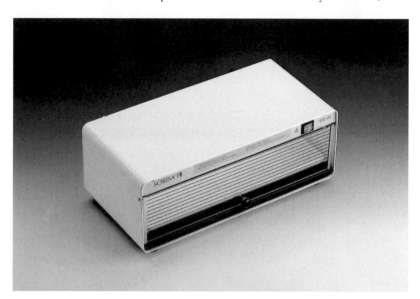

An ultraviolet cabinet

Disinfectants

These chemicals are effective only if used correctly. They quickly become stale or overloaded, and must be used at the correct concentrations for the correct length of time.

Personal hygiene and posture

Salon hygiene is extremely important, but personal hygiene is equally necessary both for yourself and for your client.

See Chapter 1 regarding personal hygiene (page 5).

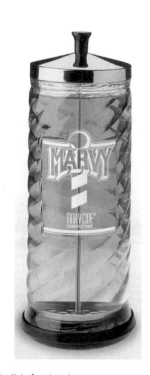

A disinfecting jar

Good posture

Good posture not only looks better, allowing clothes to hang properly, but is also more healthy because it allows the bones, muscles, tendons and ligaments to be held in their correct positions, avoiding undue stretching and strain.

Standing correctly

In order to stand correctly, keep the feet hip-width apart, with the weight of the body equally on both legs and the knees slightly bent. Hips and shoulders should be level and the head held up. Common faults are round shoulders, hollow back, and weight held mostly on one foot so that shoulders and hips are tilted.

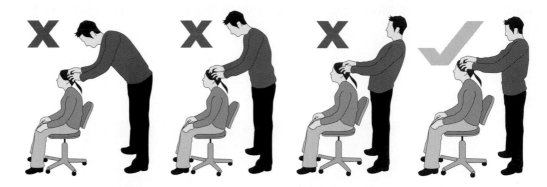

Sitting correctly

In order to sit correctly, the bones should form a right angle at the hip and knee, with the hips and most of the thighs supported by the chair. Common faults are slouching (only the base of the spine in contact with the chair so that the back and thighs are not supported) and crossing the legs.

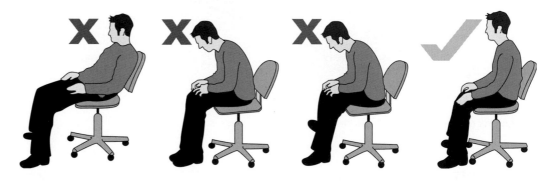

Regular exercise

All muscles need to be worked if they are to remain healthy. If under-used, muscles will begin to weaken and waste away. Regular exercise, such as running, swimming, aerobics and brisk walking will keep the muscles working correctly and help to maintain a good body shape. Exercise will also improve respiration, digestion and blood circulation, as well as relaxing nervous tension.

Safe practices in the salon

Working safely in the salon is not just a matter of common sense. There are now many government laws and Acts which are designed to protect staff, clients and the environment.

Here is a brief summary of the main laws and Acts that affect hairdressers.

The Health and Safety at Work Act 1974

Under the Act, it is the duty of every employee at work to take reasonable care not to endanger the health, safety or welfare of others. Employees must not interfere with or misuse any items provided in the interests of health and safety.

The Manual Handling Operations Regulation 1992

This states that all employees at work have a duty to minimise the risks from lifting and handling objects.

The Personal Protective Equipment at Work Regulations 1992

These regulations confirm the requirement for all employers to provide suitable and sufficient protective clothing, and for all employees to use it when required. In the case of hairdressers, this means wearing protective gloves and tinting aprons when colouring, bleaching, perming and relaxing.

The Provision and Use of Work Equipment Regulations 1992/8

Under these regulations, employers have a duty to select equipment for use at work which is properly constructed, suitable for the purpose and kept in good repair. Employers must also ensure that all who use the equipment have been adequately trained.

The requirement for competence to use salon tools and equipment is embodied within these hairdressing standards.

The Control of Substances Hazardous to Health Act 1999 (COSHH)

This is enforced by Health and Safety inspectors. It is particularly relevant to the storage and use of hazardous chemicals such as hydrogen peroxide or perm lotions.

It applies not only to you but also to chemicals applied and sold to non-employees, i.e. clients.

The Act states that staff must be given information, instruction and training on both hazardous and potentially hazardous chemicals used in the salon.

The HMWA (The Hairdressing Manufacturers' and Wholesalers' Association Ltd) publish an excellent leaflet, *A Guide to Health and Safety in the Salon*, which is available to all salons. There is also a free leaflet, *Five Steps for Completing COSHH Assessments*, which is available from your local Health and Safety Executive (HSE) office.

Fire Precautions Act 1971

This is enforced by the local fire authority, usually the fire brigade. It states that all premises must have fire-fighting equipment which is in good working order, suitable for the types of fire that are likely to occur, and readily available. It also states that room contents should be arranged and doors left unlocked to enable a quick exit in case of fire.

The Reporting of Injuries, Diseases and Dangerous Occurrences Regulations 1995 (RIDDOR)

If you, your staff or your clients suffer from a personal injury at work, it must be reported in the salon's Accident Book. This is in order to inform your employer, and so that serious injuries may be reported to the local Enforcement Office.

TO DO

It may be that you are responsible for some or all of the areas covered by these Acts. If it is not written in your job description, then ask your salon manager/owner for clarification.

Electricity at Work Regulations 1992

These state that every electrical appliance in a work site must be tested at least every 12 months by a qualified electrician. A written record must be kept of these tests, to be shown to the Health and Safety authorities upon inspection.

The Environmental Protection Act 1990

This states that hairdressing salon chemicals (i.e. 'waste') must be disposed of safely, i.e. poured down the sink (to dilute and remove them). Never put them in the dustbin where they could be found by children.

The Health and Safety (First Aid) Regulations 1981

These regulations require every employer to provide equipment and facilities appropriate for administering first aid to their employees.

Health and Safety at Work Act 1974 (HASAWA)

This is enforced by Environmental Health Officers and Health and Safety Inspectors. It protects almost everyone involved in working situations. It states the responsibilities of the employer and the employees relating to:

- First aid (emergency aid) arrangements and the reporting of accidents
- General health and safety
- Enforcement of the Act.

Penalties and fines

Failure to comply with the Health and Safety at Work Act 1974 carries the following penalties and fines:

- Minor offences, e.g. obstructing an Enforcing Officer: fines up to £5,000
- Serious offences, e.g. failing to comply with an improvement order from the Enforcing Officer: fines up to £20,000 and/or six months' imprisonment
- Very serious offences, e.g. resulting in death: unlimited fines and/or up to two years' imprisonment.

Therefore you must take health and safety seriously.

Health and safety checklist

Does your salon have five or more employees? If so, then you must have a written Health and Safety Policy as shown below.

HEALTH AND SAFETY AT WORK ACT 1974

General Statement of Policy

Our salon's policy is to provide and maintain safe and healthy working conditions, equipment and systems of work for all our employees. We will provide such information, training and supervision as is required for this purpose. We also accept our responsibility for the health and safety of clients and any other people who may be affected by our activities. We will maintain safe access to and egress from our premises at all times.

Name _____

Position _____

Date _____

Review Arrangements

This policy will need to be reviewed at least every six months and amended as required. All members of staff will be involved in the review.

The person responsible for instigating the review is:

Name _____

The Health and Safety Policy must also give details of review arrangements as shown below:

Health and Safety Policy Review Dates		
	Planned date	Actual review
1		
2		
3		
4		

Also required is a full statement of staff duties and responsibilities with regard to health and safety. An example is shown below.

Health & Safety at Work Act 1974

Statement of staff responsibilities

Overall responsibility for health and safety in the salon is that of:

Name _____

Position _____

The person responsible for health and safety on a day-to-day basis (normally you, the supervisor, or manager) in the salon is:

Name _____

Position _____

In the above person's absence, the following person will be responsible as his/her deputy:

Name _____

Position _____

The person responsible for health and safety training is:

Name _____

The person responsible for enforcing salon rules is:

Name _____

The person responsible for first aid and in particular checking the first aid box contents and re-stocking as necessary is:

Name _____

The first aid box is kept: _____

The trained and qualified first aider is:

Name _____ Type of qualification _____

Certificate number _____ Expiry date _____

The person responsible for the Accident Book and for reporting accidents is:

Name _____

The Accident Book is kept: _____

The person responsible for fire safety and in particular checking fire extinguishers, fire exit signs, escape routes and organising fire drills is:

Name _____

The person responsible for providing and replenishing personal protective equipment is:

Name _____

The person responsible for inspecting electrical equipment such as the portable hand tools on a three-monthly basis and adding any new/replacement tools to the checklist is:

Name _____

The person responsible for carrying out, updating and monitoring the COSHH assessments is:

Name _____

The COSHH assessments are kept: _____

Day-to-day responsibilities under HASAWA

You will need to know where you can access information on health and safety legislation. It may be from:

● Health and safety literature from HSE and the Hairdressing Training Board
● The local library
● Your local council offices
● Reference books.

It is also a good idea to produce a chart of key names and addresses for quick reference, e.g.:

Health and Safety Policy: Important Contacts			
Key contact	Contact name	Tel/fax	Address
Environmental Health Officer			
Hospital			
Doctor			
Fire Safety Officer			
Employment Medical Advisory Service			
Local Police Station			

Health and Safety Law

What you should know

HSE
Health & Safety
Executive

Leaflet published by the Health and Safety Executive

REMEMBER

It is a legal requirement to display the Health and Safety Law poster in your salon.

Once you have collected and itemised all your information you need to know how to pass this on to the rest of the staff. You could do this through:

● Staff meetings and verbal discussions
● Training days
● Displaying and/or circulating memos and leaflets (see Salon Rules, page 47)
● Implementing the information in the salon

- By displaying notices such as:

<table>
<tr><td>

FIRE DRILL

IN THE EVENT OF A FIRE

1. TELEPHONE 999 FOR THE FIRE BRIGADE
2. CLOSE ALL DOORS AND WINDOWS
3. LEAVE THE BUILDING BY THE NEAREST EXIT
4. ASSEMBLE OUTSIDE THE SALON

DO NOT

1. STOP TO COLLECT ANY PERSONAL BELONGINGS
2. RE-ENTER THE BUILDING UNTIL THE ALL CLEAR HAS BEEN GIVEN

THE NEAREST EXITS ARE:

THE SALON FRONT DOOR, THE SALON BACK DOOR

</td><td>

*IF YOU FIND AN UNATTENDED PARCEL, A SUSPICIOUS OBJECT, OR IF YOU SUSPECT THAT THERE IS LIKELY TO BE AN EXPLOSIVE DEVICE, GAS LEAK ETC. IN OR NEAR YOUR SALON

- DO NOT TOUCH OR MOVE THE PARCEL/OBJECT
- EVACUATE THE SALON
- CALL THE POLICE
- WARN MEMBERS OF THE PUBLIC
- WARN THE OCCUPANTS OF ADJACENT PREMISES

DO NOT RE-ENTER THE AREA UNTIL INSTRUCTED TO DO SO BY THE POLICE

ALWAYS REMEMBER
IF IN DOUBT – SHOUT!

</td></tr>
</table>

You will need to identify your salon's hazards and risks and record them by using this form:

Health and Safety Risk Evaluation					
	Potential hazard	Degree of risk Low/Med/High (please circle)	Persons at risk	Action needed to minimise risk	By when	By whom
1		L M H				
2		L M H				
3		L M H				
4		L M H				
5		L M H				

The Management of Health & Safety at Work Regulations 1992/99

This legislation requires salon owners to maintain and improve health and safety at work, provide proper training and to evaluate risk assessments.

Health and safety training

A lot of time and money is spent training someone to become a hairdresser. This would be completely wasted if they end up being unable to work as a result of poor health and safety training.

Salon Rules

Salon safety and hygiene

- Fixtures, fittings, chairs, trolleys and mirrors to be regularly cleaned.
- Non-electrical equipment to be kept clean and sterilised at all times.
- Electrical equipment to be visually checked for safety, then switched off, unplugged and stored between use.
- Floors to be swept clean, free from hair, and spillages immediately mopped up.
- Used gowns and towels to be placed in the laundry basket.
- Rubbish to be removed immediately and placed in a covered container. Store in sealed rubbish bags while awaiting disposal.
- Food and drink must be consumed only in the staff restroom.
- Restroom to be kept clean and tidy. Wash up cups, plates and saucers immediately after use.
- Staff who smoke must use the smoking area in the restroom.
- Stock room to be kept clean and tidy. Stock to be correctly stored and lids and tops replaced immediately after use.
- Reception area to be kept clean and tidy.

Fire precautions

- Smoking is only allowed in designated areas of the salon and outside the back entrance.
- Keep all fire exits and egress to them clear at all times.
- Do not obstruct fire extinguishers.
- Unlock fire exits during working hours.

Security

- Keep till drawer locked when not in use.
- Keep all stock doors and cupboards locked when not in use.
- Do not bring any valuables to the salon. Keep your purse/money on your person at all times.
- Lock all fire exits, close all windows and lock all doors at night.

Basic health and safety induction should be carried out on the first day the employee or trainee starts work and completed by the end of the first week. The induction should cover the following:

- **The salon's Health and Safety Policy.** Give the person a copy of the Health and Safety Law leaflet (see page 45) and point out the Key Names and Addresses chart. If you display a Health and Safety law poster, then explain this to them. Also give them a copy of the Salon Rules.

- **Fire precautions.** Explain where the fire extinguishers are kept and how to use them. Point out the fire drill notices and show them where the nearest fire exits are. Tell them who is responsible for fire safety. Note that fire extinguishers colour-coded blue (dry powder), black (CO_2) and green (vaporising liquids) can be used on electrical fires. Red (water, CO_2, soda acid) and cream (foam) must **never** be used on electrical fires – water conducts electricity and you will be electrocuted.

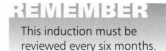

REMEMBER

This induction must be reviewed every six months.

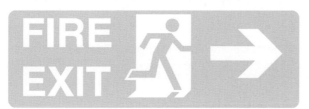

These signs are now mandatory

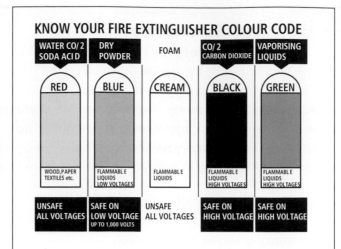

Fire extinguisher codes

- **First-aid arrangements.** Tell them who is responsible for first aid in the salon and show them where the first-aid box is kept (see page 59). Explain who is responsible for the reporting of accidents and the Accident Book.

- **COSHH.** Outline the COSHH Act 1988 to them and tell them who is responsible for carrying out, updating and monitoring the COSHH assessments.

- **Personal protective equipment.** Show them where the gloves and aprons are kept and tell them when they should be used.

- **Electrical equipment.** Tell them who is responsible for inspecting electrical equipment and what to do if they notice anything that looks dangerous.

- **Contingency precautions.** Show them where the main electricity switch, the water stopcock and the main gas valve are located.

Keep a record of all staff health and safety inductions and reviews, e.g.:

Staff name	Signature	Date	Areas inducted								Health and safety review dates			
			Health & safety policy and salon rules	Fire precautions	First aid and accidents	COSSH	Personal protective equipment	Electrical equipment	Trainer's signature				

Health and Safety Training Record

To make sure that the member of staff has understood the induction, ask them to complete the following questionnaire:

The Manual Handling Regulations 1992

These regulations cover the lifting of loads such as salon stock or video units, as well as lowering, pushing, pulling, carrying and moving them, whether by hand or by using bodily force.

To prevent accidents and injuries when lifting, you should bear in mind the following:

- **The weight of the load.** Try to use a trolley to transport heavy or bulky items into the dispensary and stock rooms. If the package is too heavy for you, either ask another member of staff to help you or unpack the box carefully until it is light enough to be moved.
- **The shape of the load.** Some loads may not be particularly heavy but are bulky and awkward to lift.
- **Distribution of load.** Before attempting to lift, look inside boxes to ensure that the contents are evenly distributed.
- **Your personal limitations.** If you have recently had an illness such as flu, you may not have regained your normal strength.
- **Loose items.** Check for loose staples before attempting to lift boxes, and do not put loose items on top of the box when lifting.
- **The working environment.** If the area is damp, your hands could be wet and the load might slip.
- **Ease of access.** Will you have to negotiate awkward doorways or stairs?
- **Storage.** Sometimes stock needs to be stored on high shelves. Always use a strong, sturdy stepladder, never a chair or anything unsteady.

Lifting heavy loads

When lifting, keep your knees bent and your back straight at all times. If you lift incorrectly you could strain a ligament or damage a joint in your spine.

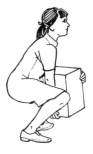
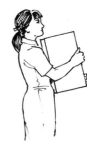

Always lift heavy loads with knees bent and back straight

- Keep your feet apart, one foot slightly in front of the other to maintain your balance, and face the direction in which the object is to be moved. Never try to lift in a sideways direction.
- Grip the package firmly, keeping it close to your body with your chin tucked well in. Keep the package close to your body, bending at your knees and hips and making sure that your knees are directly above your feet. Allow your strong leg muscles to take the weight, not your back.
- When lowering the object to the ground, be careful to keep your back straight, feet apart and knees and hips bent. Gently does it: remember that lowering heavy objects can be just as dangerous as lifting them.

There are five main types of injury that can occur due to manual handling:
- Disc injuries
- Muscular/nerve injuries
- Ligament/tendon injuries
- Hernias
- Fractures, abrasions and cuts.

These can all be avoided by observing the above procedure.

The major risk in a salon is from lifting boxes of stock items onto and off shelves. The risk assessment in this case is a very simple one and, although it needs to be carried out, it need not be formally recorded.

Personal Protective Equipment at Work Regulations 1992

The requirements of these regulations will have been met when you comply with your COSHH regulations.

The regulations require employers to provide suitable protective clothing for all employees to use when required. This includes, for example, wearing protective gloves and tinting aprons when colouring, bleaching, perming and relaxing.

Staff must be trained and monitored to ensure that these regulations are properly enforced.

The Provision and Use of Work Equipment Regulations 1992

The following requirements apply to all equipment from 1 January 1993:
- Work equipment must be suitable for the purpose for which it is used.
- All equipment must be properly maintained and records kept.
- All salon staff must be given adequate health and safety training and written instructions where required.

TO DO

Complete the following checklist, ticking if the answer is Yes, taking appropriate action if the answer is No.

- *Is all the equipment in my salon regularly checked to make sure that it is in serviceable condition?*
- *Do I keep maintenance records, particularly for electrical equipment?*
- *Is second-hand equipment checked by a competent person before use?*
- *Have all staff been trained in the safe use of all salon equipment?*

Electricity at Work Regulations 1992

These regulations cover the installation, maintenance and use of electrical systems and equipment.

The salon's electrical circuits and all electrical equipment should be tested at least every 12 months by a qualified electrician. Each electrical hand tool should be listed, numbered and marked with the last test date.

Schedule of Electrical Items			
Item	Serial no.	Purchase date	Disposal date
1			
2			
3			
4			

Regular safety precautions should include:

- Removing any trailing electrical cables (dry flexes).
- Checking the temperature controls before using any equipment, and making sure the filters at the back of hairdriers are clear and free of dust to prevent overheating.
- Always switching off and disconnecting equipment straight after use.
- Clear labelling of any faulty electrical equipment, which should also be reported.

In addition, a three-monthly visual check on hand tools should be carried out by a member of staff. This should include:

- Looking at equipment to make sure that flexes and cables are not worn or faulty. Any flexes with worn insulation or any plugs that are broken or cracked should be replaced.
- Making sure that electrical equipment is stable. Check that hairdriers, tongs or hot brushes are safely stored on the work surface and not in places where they are likely to fall off.

Electric shock

This occurs when a person's body completes an electrical circuit. The size of the shock depends on the size of the electrical current, and can vary from a slight tingling to a cardiac arrest (when the heart stops beating and breathing stops).

> **REMEMBER**
>
> All tools brought in by members of staff must be numbered, added to the list of items in the Electrical Equipment Register and included in the checks along with any new equipment purchased.

> **REMEMBER**
>
> E = EARTH = green and yellow wire
> N = NEUTRAL = blue wire
> L = LIVE = brown wire

Testing Programme for Salon Appliances							
ELECTRICAL SUPPLIER			TESTING DATES				
Name and address	Tel. No.	Target	Actual	Target	Actual	Target	Actual

It can happen when a person touches bare wires on flexes or cables, through incorrect wiring or a fault in the plug or appliance, or as a result of touching a switch or plug with wet hands (water acts as a conductor and electricity will flow through the person rather than through the circuit).

Wiring a plug

It is strongly recommended that a residual current device, known as an earth leakage trip, rated at 30mA, be fitted in the circuits to which hand tools are connected. Make sure you know how to wire a plug correctly:

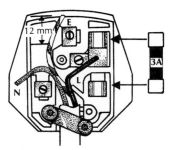

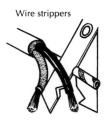

1 Cut away the outer cable, unscrew the cable grip and insert the cable

2 Cut away the insulation using wire strippers

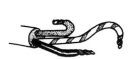

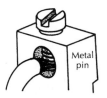

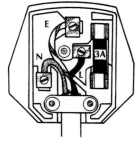

3 Twist the copper strands together

4 Insert each wire into the correct pin

5 Tighten all the screws and the cable grip. Attach the plastic back

The Control of Substances Hazardous to Health Act 1988 (COSHH)

Chemical substances are hazardous as a result of:

- **Inhalation** – breathing in fumes
- **Ingestion** – swallowing them directly or by eating food while chemicals are on the fingers
- **Absorption** – through the skin or via the eyes

- **Contact** – with the skin or eye surface (a chemical of this sort is known as an irritant)
- Being **injected** into the body
- Being introduced into the body via **cuts**, etc.

Basic safety rules for storage of salon chemicals are as follows:
- Never use food or drink containers to store any chemical product
- Store products at or below room temperature in a dry atmosphere, never in direct sunlight, and according to manufacturers' instructions
- Store all glass bottles below eye level
- Keep products, particularly aerosols, away from naked flames or heat
- Take special care to prevent children gaining access to salon storage areas. Keep all products out of the reach of children.

Mixing chemicals safely

- Follow the manufacturer's instructions exactly
- Dilute the product according to the manufacturer's recommendations
- Never mix products unless this is recommended by the manufacturer
- Replace all caps and bottletops immediately to avoid spillage. Make sure unused mixtures and empty containers are disposed of carefully.

Using chemicals safely

- Always wear protective gloves and protective clothing where indicated (see chart on page 54). Remember that prolonged and frequent use of non-hazardous products such as shampoos may cause dryness and sore skin. To avoid this, wear protective gloves or use barrier cream and moisturiser as often as possible
- Wipe and clean all surfaces where spillages occur. Under the COSHH regulations employers must:
  - Identify substances in the workplace which are potentially hazardous
  - Keep records of manufacturers' data sheets for all chemicals and products and carefully assess any new chemicals and products before use
- Assess the risk to health from exposure to hazardous substances and record the results
- Assess which members of staff are at risk
- Look for alternative, less hazardous substances and substitute these if possible
- Decide what precautions are required, noting that personal protective equipment should be provided free of charge
- Introduce effective measures to prevent or control exposure to potentially hazardous substances
- Inform, instruct and train all members of staff
- Review the assessment on a regular basis.

See the table showing Chemical Hazards and Precautions, page 54.

Ask staff to find out how to:
- *Operate the salon's heating system through the use of thermostats*
- *Ventilate the salon by opening the windows or using the extractor fans.*

Controlling the salon environment

This means making sure that the salon does not become too hot or cold and is well ventilated to protect against dangerous fumes.

The Health and Safety at Work Act 1974 states that the working temperature should be 16°C (60.8°F) after the first hour. Precautions should also be taken to avoid salons becoming humid due to hair-drying equipment and steam from hot water supplies, which can also make for difficult working conditions.

Ventilation

The COSHH regulations also cover ventilation, especially when mixing chemicals (think about the smell when mixing powder bleach, for instance), so make sure products are mixed in a well-ventilated area.

CHEMICAL HAZARDS AND PRECAUTIONS

Chemicals	Health hazard	Precautions
All aerosols, including hairspray	Dangerous if inhaled excessively	Use in a well-ventilated area. Keep well away from lit cigarettes
	Flammable	Do not tamper with valves: the contents are under pressure and can explode in a fire
Setting lotions, mousses and gels	Potential irritant	Avoid eye contact
	Flammable	Keep away from lit cigarettes
Hydrogen peroxide	Irritant to skin and eyes	Always wear protective gloves
		Avoid contacts with eyes and sensitive skin
		Replace cap immediately after use
		Do not allow to mix with other chemicals as it can react and become explosive
Bleaches	Dangerous if inhaled excessively	Use in a well-ventilated area
	Irritant to skin and eyes	Wear protective gloves
		Avoid contact with eyes and sensitive skin
Perm lotions and relaxers	Irritant to skin and eyes	Wear protective gloves
		Avoid contact with eyes and sensitive skin
Perm neutralisers	Irritant to skin and eyes	Wear protective gloves
		Avoid contact with eyes and sensitive skin
Hair colours, tints and semi-permanents	Irritant to skin and eyes	Wear protective gloves
	Can cause allergic reactions	Avoid contact with eyes and sensitive skin
		Always do a skin test before use

COSSH Risk Assessment							
Hazard	What is the risk?	Degree of risk			Who is at risk?	Action to be taken	Date
		High	Med	Low			

Remember also that portable gas or paraffin heaters need proper ventilation to prevent any build-up of irritant gases.

Fire Precautions Act 1971

Under this Act, a fire certificate is required for the premises if:

- More than 20 people are employed on one floor at any one time
- More than 10 people are employed on different floors at any one time.

If the premises are shared with other employers, you must include all people working in the premises when deciding if a fire certificate is required. If your salon is rented or leased, always check with the landlord if a fire certificate is required and if so, find out whether a certificate has already been issued. Check with the local fire brigade if you have any doubts.

Whether or not a fire certificate is required, **all** premises must be provided with an adequate means of escape and appropriate fire-fighting equipment.

Fire drill notices explaining what to do in case of fire must be clearly displayed. All fire exits should be clearly marked with the appropriate signs.

Staff should not use fire extinguishers unless they have been fully trained in their use.

Emergency procedures

You must know how to vacate your building quickly and safely in the case of fire, flood, gas leaks, suspicious packages or a bomb alert, and be able to locate the assembly points outside the salon. You must be aware of where fire-fighting equipment is kept and trained staff must know how to use it.

TO DO

Use the COSHH Risk Assessments chart above to assess your salon's risks.

REMEMBER

Fire in the salon may be caused by:
- Incorrect handling of inflammable hairdressing chemicals, such as ethyl acetate (nail polish remover) and hairspray
- Careless cigarette smoking.

Fire Equipment Test Record							
FIRE EQUIPMENT SUPPLIER		TESTING DATES					
Name and address	Tel. No.	Target	Actual	Target	Actual	Target	Actual

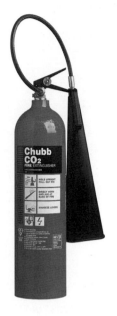

Fire extinguisher

The Environmental Protection Act 1990

Under this Act, anyone disposing of waste chemicals has a duty of care to ensure all the waste is disposed of safely.

For the purposes of the Act, all of the salon's chemicals are considered to be waste. They must therefore be diluted for disposal – i.e. poured down the sink – thereby lessening their potential adverse effects on the environment.

It is important to take care when disposing of surplus or out-of-date stock. Always check with the manufacturers for guidance. If in doubt, ask the manufacturer to dispose of the stock for you.

The Reporting of Injuries, Diseases and Dangerous Occurrences Regulations 1995 (RIDDOR)

These regulations require that if you or your staff suffer personal injury at work resulting in:

1. A fatality
2. A major injury
3. More than 24 hours in hospital
4. Incapacity for more than three calendar days (excluding the day of injury but including weekends and holidays)

the incident must be notified in writing to the local Enforcement Officer.

This is done by completing form F2508 (copies of which can be obtained from either Dillons Bookshops or direct from HSE books). It should be sent within seven days of the accident or injury occurring.

If a client or visiting member of the public should suffer serious injury and be taken to hospital, or die on the premises, this must also be reported.

Notifying the Enforcement Officer

For accidents in categories 1–3 above and dangerous occurrences (e.g. a serious fire), the local Enforcement Officer must be notified quickly by telephone. This should then be followed up by form F2508.

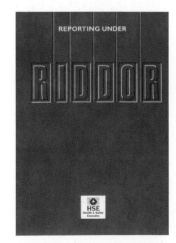

RIDDOR booklet published by the Health and Safety Executive

In addition, if a client or visitor to your premises suffers personal injury in categories 1–2 above, this must also be reported to the local Enforcement Officer.

Below is a list of salon services, possible damage and ways of avoiding that damage.

POTENTIAL CLIENT INJURY

Client service	Possible injury or damage	Precautions
Styling	Burnt skin or scalp during drying	Learn how to work drying equipment
	Damage to clothes from products	Gown the client, covering all clothes
Cutting	Cut skin	Advise client how to sit during cutting
Colouring and lightening	Allergic skin or scalp reaction	Carry out a skin test
	Hair condition deteriorating	Follow manufacturer's instructions for selection, preparation, development times and removal of products
	Hair breakage	
	Scalp burns	Gown the client, covering all clothes
	Damage to clothes from products	
Perming and relaxing	Hair condition deterioratin.	Carry out any necessary pre-treatment tests
	Hair breakage	Follow manufacturer's instructions for selection, preparation, development times and removal of products
	Scalp burns	
		Ensure correct selection of tools and equipment
		Use barrier cream

Recording accidents

All salon accidents must be reported in the salon's Accident Book. This should be set out as shown on page 58.

It is important to record **all** accidents so that when a review of health and safety procedures is carried out (which should include a review of the Accident Book) repetitions can be avoided.

Occupational dermatitis and **asthma** are also reportable. You may wish to use the following chart for your records:

TO DO

- *Ask your product suppliers for advice on the safe disposal of your chemicals and products.*
- *Check to ensure that all staff know how to dispose of chemicals and products safely.*
- *Check that all your waste products are kept in a safe place away from children.*

Asthma/Dermatitis Records				
Name	Date symptoms reported	Description of symptoms	Date of medical advice	Precautions required

TO DO

- *Remind your staff that all accidents must be recorded in the Accident Book.*
- *Check that you have copies of form F2508 available for reporting accidents.*
- *Ask staff regularly if they have signs of dermatitis or asthma. If signs of either are detected, then you must take suitable action to minimise the problem, either by providing barrier cream and gloves, or by improving ventilation and seeking medical help.*

REMEMBER

The key reason for carrying out an accident investigation is to prevent a re-occurrence – not to decide who is to blame.

Accident Book					
When did the accident happen? (Give date and time)	Where did the accident happen?	How did the accident happen? (Give as much detail as possible)	Name of person(s) involved and nature of injuries	Who investigated and reported the accident? (Give full name and position)	Was the accident reportable under RIDDOR?

First aid

REMEMBER

RIDDOR states that all accidents must be reported in the accident register kept in the salon.

Emergency aid in the salon usually involves the treatment of minor accidental injuries. However, a qualified first aider would also be able to help with more serious injuries, such as bone fractures or heart attacks, before the patient is seen by a doctor. The aim of first aid is to prevent death or further damage to injured persons. If you have any doubt about an injury, always seek medical advice from a doctor or nurse at a health clinic or the casualty department at your local hospital.

A table of common accidents and conditions in the salon is shown below.

COMMON ACCIDENTS AND CONDITIONS IN THE SALON	
Accident/condition	Emergency procedure
Salon chemicals in the eye, e.g. perm lotions, bleaches, tints.	Wash the eye with running water (under the tap if possible). Continue applying water to the eye until medical assistance is available.
Salon chemicals on the skin, e.g. perm lotions, bleach.	Flood the area with water to dilute and remove the chemical.
Salon chemicals swallowed, e.g. chemicals placed in soft-drink containers and drunk by mistake.	Drink 2–3 glasses of water. Seek medical advice immediately.
Salon chemicals inhaled, e.g. strong bleach mixtures.	Move the person to fresh air immediately. Seek medical advice if coughing, choking or breathlessness lasts longer than 10–15 minutes.
Dry heat burns, e.g. from hairdriers, tongs, hot brushes, crimping irons.	Hold affected area under running cold water or apply ice pack (5–10 minutes). Seek medical advice if necessary.
Scalds, e.g. from hot water supplies or steamers.	Hold affected area under running cold water or apply ice pack (5–10 minutes). Seek medical advice if necessary.
Minor cuts.	Apply pressure until bleeding stops. Avoid direct contact with blood because of the risk of infectious diseases such as AIDS and Hepatitis B. Wherever possible, ask clients to use a clean piece of cotton wool and apply pressure themselves, then dispose of the cotton wool in a plastic bag or bin.
Severe cuts.	The blood flow from severe cuts should be stopped by applying pressure with either a clean towel or hands (covered with rubber gloves from the first-aid box). Phone for an ambulance immediately.
Electric shock.	If someone is being electrocuted do not touch them as you will be electrocuted yourself. Turn off the electricity immediately, either by turning off the switches or pulling out the plug. If breathing has stopped then artificial respiration will need to be given by a qualified first aider. Phone for an ambulance straight away.
Client distress, e.g. fainting.	This is caused by lack of oxygen to the brain. If someone feels faint, put their head between their knees and loosen any tight clothing. If the person has fainted, raise their legs on a cushion so that they are higher than the head.

First-aid kits

All salons should provide a first-aid box (usually coloured green with a white cross) containing a first-aid kit. It should include a list of contents, plus the following:

- A first-aid guidance card
- Individually wrapped sterile adhesive dressings

- Medium, large and extra large sterile unmedicated dressings
- Sterile bandages (including a triangular bandage)
- Sterile eye pads, with attachment
- Scissors
- Tweezers
- Safety pins
- Saline lotion.

TO DO

- *Find out if your staff know where the first-aid kit is located in your salon.*
- *Check the contents to see if anything is missing, or if there are any items which should not be there, e.g. medicines.*

It is also advisable to keep disposable rubber or plastic gloves for dealing with wounds that are bleeding or weeping. Except in an emergency, aid should not be given without wearing these gloves because of the risk of AIDS and Hepatitis B.

More serious signs of distress, such as heart attacks, stopped breathing, epileptic fits or fractures (from falls) should be dealt with by a qualified first aider. If you wish to qualify, contact your local St John's Ambulance Brigade who regularly run courses.

TEST YOUR KNOWLEDGE

1 What is emergency aid?

2 When would a qualified first aider be needed?

3 When would you need to seek medical advice or call an ambulance?

4 What items would you expect to find in a first-aid box?

5 State which colour codes of fire extinguishers can be used on:
- electrical fires
- non-electrical fires

and describe why this is important.

6 If perm lotion accidentally ran into your client's eye, what would you do?

7 How would you deal with a child who has accidentally swallowed some hydrogen peroxide?

8 If some bleach spills on to your client's neck, how would you remove it?

9 What is the best treatment for someone who is choking after inhaling a strong chemical?

10 What could cause a dry heat burn?

11 How should you treat a scald on the hand caused by boiling water?

12 If you accidentally cut your client's ear, how should the bleeding be stopped?

13 Why must you always wear gloves when treating a person with a severe cut?

14 What is the most important action to take if someone is being electrocuted?

15 Why is it important to raise a person's feet if they have fainted?

Failing to comply

The consequences of your failing to comply with health and safety requirements are serious. They include:

- Harming yourself, other staff or clients
- Notice being given by the Health and Safety Office for you to implement action
- Possible legal action.

Non-compliance with health and safety requirements could be corrected by:

- Informing your manager or salon owner
- Correcting the compliance yourself if it is within your responsibility to do so
- Warning other people in order to avoid accidents whilst the matter is being dealt with.

Routine health and safety checks

The following is a list of typical health and safety checks to be carried out in the salon.

Routine Health and Safety Checks									
Inspection items/area	Staff member responsible	Inspection dates/initials							
Safety inspections									
Enforcing salon rules									
Inspecting electrical equipment									
First-aid kit									
Accident book									
Fire exits/extinguishers/fire drills									
Day-to-day health and safety inspections									
COSHH assessments									

TO DO

- *Find out exactly what your limits of authority are when dealing with non-compliance with health and safety regulations by your manager.*

TEST YOUR KNOWLEDGE

1 Describe how the following health and safety legislation affects your work role and the staff for whom you are responsible:

- The Health and Safety at Work Act 1974
- The Manual Handling Operations Regulations 1992
- The Personal Protective Equipment at Work Regulations 1992
- The Provision and Use of Work Equipment Regulations 1992
- Control of Substances Hazardous to Health Regulations 1988 (COSHH).

2 Where can you access information on the above Acts?

3 How could you pass this information on to your staff?

4 What are the potential consequences if you did not adhere to health and safety requirements?

5 How could you correct non-compliance with health and safety requirements?

6 What records must be kept with regards to:

- Health and safety checks
- Accidents
- COSHH risk assessments?

7 Describe the potential client injury or damage that could result from the following salon services, and ways of avoiding that damage:

- Styling
- Cutting
- Colouring and lighting
- Perming and relaxing.

Chapter 3 Creative cutting for men and women

Keeping up to date with the latest techniques and cutting skills is paramount to the successful hairdresser today. The profile of British hairdressing is at an all-time high and there are many great hairdressers in our industry to follow. Magazines, shows, seminars and even television highlight the skills used in cutting the wide variety of styles worn in the high street and on the catwalk.

This chapter covers the following NVQ level 3 units:
H27 Create a variety of looks using a combination of cutting techniques
H21 Create a variety of looks using a combination of barbering techniques
H22 Design and create patterns in hair.

Designing a hairstyle

When choosing a hairstyle, hairdressers will usually work under three broad categories:

- **Classic** – i.e. the more timeless styles such as bob shapes or short back and sides
- **Current** – those that are currently 'in vogue'
- **Emerging fashion** – the forerunners of fashion.

A hairstyle should be designed to suit each individual client and a good stylist should be able to adapt a style to suit any client.

Many factors may influence your choice of style. These include:

- **Client personality, lifestyle and dress.** A client who is sporty or has a hectic lifestyle will need a style that is easy to manage and requires minimum styling.
- **Age of client.** Never assume that an older client will want an old-fashioned hairstyle.
- **Body shape and size.** The chosen style must be in proportion with the body.
- **Face shape and features.** The style should be designed to suit the face shape and enhance, or disguise, facial features.

TO DO

Put together a portfolio of classic, current and emerging fashion styles.

TO DO

List the four main face shapes and think of some features that:
- may need disguising
- should be emphasised.

Client consultation

Carrying out a **thorough** consultation with the client before commencing, using style books if desired, will give both the stylist and the client a clear picture of what is to be done.

Checking with the client as the cut progresses is also a good idea as this allows any necessary adjustments or changes to be made. Consulting with your client before and during the cutting process will help to prevent any problems from arising and promote a professional image of the salon. It will also help to ensure client satisfaction. If clients feel that you have not only produced a good result but have also been attentive, listened to their concerns and given good advice, they will be encouraged to return to the salon and may even promote the salon and its services to their friends.

HEALTH MATTERS

Remember to check hair and scalp for any contagious disorders during your consultation. Failure to recognise potential infections or infestations could result in infecting yourself and others (cross-infection).

The hair

As well as client limitations, the hair itself must be considered before deciding on a style. Each of the following will influence the style and cutting techniques chosen:

- Thickness/density
- Texture
- Length – short, medium, long
- Condition and quality – remember to carry out porosity and elasticity tests
- Hair type – European, African Caribbean, Asian
- Hair growth patterns – cowlick, nape whorl, widow's peak, male pattern baldness, scarring
- Existing body or curl – curly, wavy, straight.

By paying attention to these influencing factors you will be able to create a hairstyle which will maximise the potential of the client's hair, producing the best possible result and creating a style which not only suits the client but also complements their lifestyle, appearance and personality. Ways of enhancing the haircut include the addition of colour and perming services or even adding hair to areas where thinning is apparent. Colouring techniques can be used to enhance the look of the haircut, for example a semi/quasi colour can be applied to give shine and gloss to a sleek bob or slices/strands of hair can be coloured to give definition and emphasise particular areas of a haircut. Some styles may need additional curl, body or root movement, which can be provided by perming, in order to recreate a specific look or to make the style easier for the client to manage at home. Added hair comes in a variety of products – this is widely covered in the next chapter.

Preparation of client

Always gown up the client with a cutting gown that totally covers their clothing so as to protect it from water and hair cuttings. In many salons a cutting collar is used in place of a towel to keep the neck free from obstruction when cutting. When using clippers a strip of cotton wool can be put under the neck of the gown to catch any hair clippings.

A note on facial and ear piercings
Check for facial and ear piercings, ask the client to remove as many as they can so you don't catch them with your comb. Fresh piercings should be covered with a plaster to protect them from hair clippings which could cause an infection.

Preparation of tools and equipment

Make sure that all cutting tools and equipment are clean and sterilised before use and that equipment is positioned for ease of use but is out of the reach of any children in the salon. When using electric clippers always make a visual check of cables, plugs and switches before use and remember to turn off the power supply after use.

Health and safety when cutting

Health and safety are very important when cutting hair. When handling cutting tools, avoid accidents by:

- Never carrying cutting tools in pockets
- Taking care when replacing and using open-blade razors
- Keeping cutting tools in protective cases when not in use
- Keeping sharp tools out of the reach of children
- Learning how to use each piece of cutting equipment correctly
- Cleaning and sterilising equipment after use
- Storing them safely in an allocated area.

TO DO

Find out your salon and local authority procedures for the disposal of used razor blades (sharps) and why it is important to dispose of them correctly.

Accidents when cutting

Accidentally cutting the client
If an accident does happen, keep calm and give the client a sterile dressing; ask them to apply this to the cut with pressure to stop bleeding. Do not touch the cut yourself because of health risks such as AIDS and Hepatitis B. Small cuts may be covered with a sterile dressing but larger cuts may need medical attention.

REMEMBER

Sweep up hair cuttings immediately and place in a covered bin to prevent accidents and the risk of cross-infection.

REMEMBER

Keeping your work area clean and tidy will show a professional image to clients/potential clients, promote effective and efficient working practices and help to prevent the risk of cross-infection.

Accidentally cutting yourself

Many hairdressers cut themselves during hair cutting. Stop whatever you are doing and excuse yourself from the client. Rinse the cut with water to remove any hairs, then apply pressure with a sterile dressing until the blood clots and bleeding stops. Dry the area and apply a sterile plaster.

Cleaning cutting equipment

Metal cutting tools can be cleaned by wiping with cotton wool and **surgical spirit** to disinfect them. They can also be sterilised in an **ultraviolet cabinet**. Liquid disinfectants are not advisable as prolonged use can cause the metal to become corroded. An **autoclave** can also be used.

The cut

Because cutting is a creative process it is not possible to have rules for every haircut. Stylists develop their own style of working, but each haircut must be controlled.

The cut is controlled by:

- **Accurate guidelines**. The first cut in each section determines the length for the rest of the section. Guidelines must be followed for an even haircut.
- **Correct angles of hair to the head**. Many angles may be used when cutting the hair. They will affect the shape and balance of the cut.
- **Correct angle of cut**. Many angles can be used, depending on the chosen style. They will also affect the shape, balance and length of the hairstyle.
- **Clean and neat sectioning**. This will make sure no meshes are missed and that you work in a neat, methodical way, which gives a more professional appearance and result. Some hairdressers like to use products in the hair while they are cutting because this sometimes makes sectioning and controlling the hair easier.

Baselines

Many hairstyles have clearly defined **perimeter**, or **outer**, design lines. Within these design lines the hair may be **one length**, **graduated** or **layered** and a variety of lengths. Many styles are based on variations of the following design lines. Different effects can be created depending on:

- The **angle** they are used in relation to the head
- The **combination** of one or more lines
- The **type, texture and density** of the hair.

TO DO

Ask your supervisor or product representative which products are suitable to use when cutting.

Straight baseline

Hair is cut to a horizontal line, producing an even result (below left).

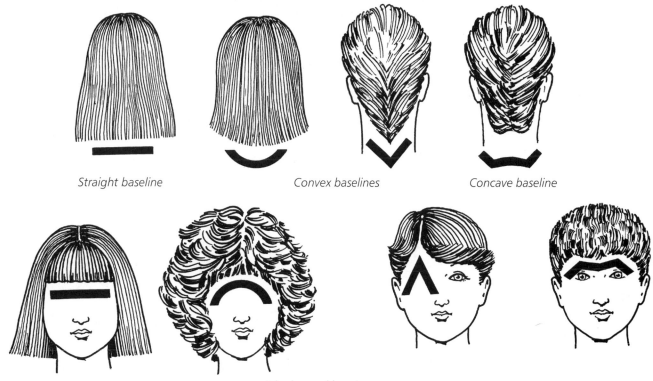

Straight baseline   *Convex baselines*   *Concave baseline*

Fringing and layering

Convex baseline

Hair is cut so that the centre back section is cut longer than the sides (above centre). A steep angle will encourage hair to fall from the shortest point to the longest point, whereas a soft curve will produce a 'U' shape if used at the nape.

Concave baselines

The hair is cut so that the centre back section is shorter than the sides (above right). An inverted 'V' will push hair away from its central, shortest point, whereas a soft curve, when used at the nape of the neck, will give a straight line – this is often used to give an even result when cutting hair with a nape whorl.

These lines can also be used when cutting fringes or when layering the hair to produce different results (when fashion styling).

Back hairlines for men

Normal hairlines that grow down may be cut either square or round by using the scissors or the clippers turned over, depending on the client's requirements. Generally, an uneven hairline is best left longer so that the hair can be cut evenly around it.

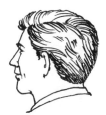
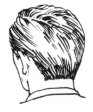
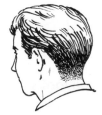

Round neckline   *Square neckline*   *Tapered neckline*

Male pattern baldness or receding hairlines generally suit a shorter haircut, rather than having a long piece of hair trailing over the top – but use good communication skills here before cutting it off – the client may like it.

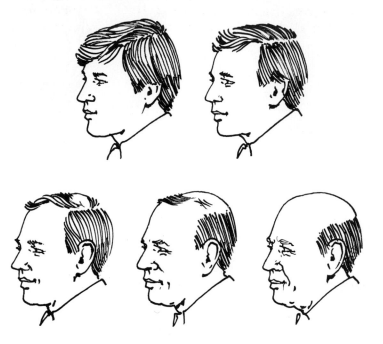

REMEMBER

Always check for the presence of added hairpieces, such as a toupe, before you start cutting.

Cicatrical alopecia or scarring, where the hair does not grow, should not be exposed – leave the hair longer to cover over.

Layering

There are many different forms of layering. Listed below are the most popular methods.

1. Basic layer

The basic layer method produces layers that are of an even length throughout the head by holding sections at a 90° angle from the head during the hair cut.

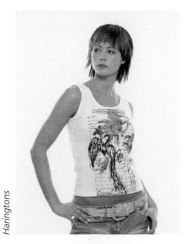

Haringtons

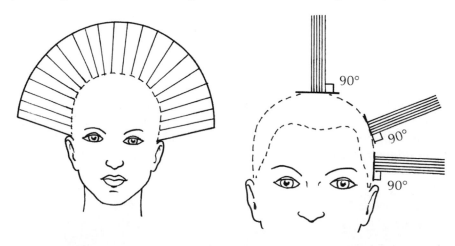

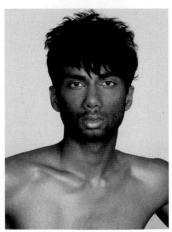

Headmasters

2. Short layered looks

Technically, a man's haircut does not need to match perfectly in the way that a woman's haircut does. It is judged visually, i.e. the finished outline shape must look perfect.

3. High/increase layering

Sometimes called high graduation, this method produces shorter layers through the top and crown area, becoming longer through the back and sides. This is achieved by holding top sections at 90° and increasing this to 180° as you progress to the back and side sections by **over-directing** (pulling hair upwards) to meet the shorter layers. See colour plate 1.

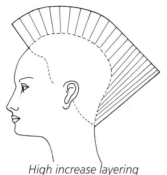

High increase layering

4. Graduation

This method gives a style in which the inner layers are longer than the outline shape. Once a guideline has been cut (usually at the hairline), sections are held at 45° from the head, either vertically or horizontally, and cut to create graduation. See colour plates 1–2.

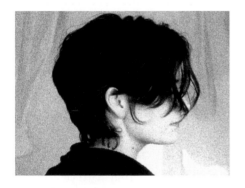

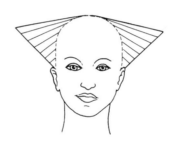

Reverse graduation

5. Reverse graduation

Used when cutting hair to one length. Once the initial guideline has been cut, each subsequent section is cut slightly longer, allowing the hair to turn under easily. This technique is often used when cutting a bob.

6. Disconnection

This cutting technique should only be used by very well-practised hairdressers for fashion styles and is also used for putting shorter layers into long hair without losing the heaviness at the bottom. In thick hair, taper cutting would be used to blend the two sections. (See the front cover.)

Men's styles

Styles without a parting
These may be worn:

- back off the face
- forwards onto the face
- brushed across to either side.

REMEMBER

Always protect the ears during cutting by covering with either your comb or your hand.

The cutting is always the same on top – i.e. it is held at 90° and perfectly even when checked in every direction.

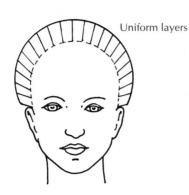

Uniform layers

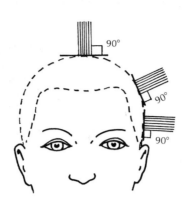

90°

90°

90°

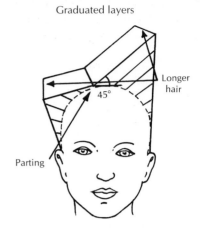

Graduated layers

Longer hair

45°

Parting

Styles with a parting

These normally have longer hair on either side of the parting to weigh the hair down. The hair is over-directed and held at 45°, not 90°, to create the length. The longer length weight line is created first and then the shorter layers are held at 45° and blended in to match.

Styles without a fringe

In these styles the hair is worn either back off the face or over to the side.

Styles with a fringe

These are when the hair is styled forward onto the face. To cut the hair with or without a fringe the front hair may be the same length as the top or a little longer, but still matching the layers.

The longer front hair is needed for blow drying back into a 'quiff' or 50s style, or if the fringe needs to cover a high forehead. Always texturise or 'chip into' (chipping is the same as pointing) the ends of a fringe to create softness on a man's haircut.

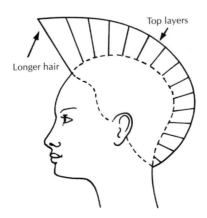

Top layers

Longer hair

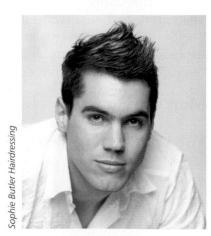

Sophie Butler Hairdressing

Styles with ears exposed

In such styles the hair is cut around the ear against the natural hairline. Always look at the distance between this hairline and the ears – there should not be a large gap or space. If the natural hairline is higher than the ears leave the hair a little longer to reduce the gap. Check the length of the sides with your client – does he want sideburns, a straight line or a pointed shape?

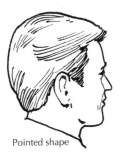 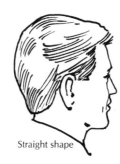 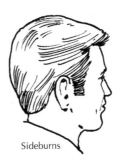

Pointed shape   Straight shape   Sideburns

Once you have created the shape you may have to remove any unwanted hair with an open razor. Remember to check in the mirror to see that the sideburns are level at both sides.

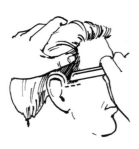 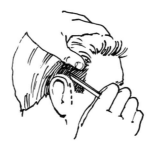

TO DO

● *Find four different photographs of men's short haircuts.*
● *Make brief notes on the cutting and layering techniques.*
● *Ask your supervisor to comment on your work.*

Styles where the ears are covered

These also need careful cutting. Never pull the hair tight or use tension over the ears because the hair will lift up and become shorter when you let go! Just comb the hair evenly and cut it freehand to achieve the correct length.

Cutting techniques using scissors

Scissors

Most hairdressers use 11.5–12.75 cm (4.5–5 in.) scissors for cutting women's hair, and use only 1.25 cm (half an inch) of the blade for cutting. Men's haircuts often take about 20 minutes, and therefore you need longer blades (14–15.25 cm or 5.5–6 in.) to cut more quickly.

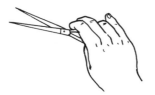

Club cutting

This is the most common cutting technique. However, it must be precise and is often called **precision cutting**. The sub-section of hair must be cleanly combed through and held with an even tension before cutting.

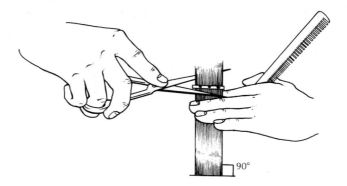

The diagram shows hair cut at 90° for a layer cut, but the hair may be cut at any angle to the head according to the style planned. Club cutting may be done on wet or dry hair and the ends of the hair are left blunt and heavy (this is sometimes also called **blunt cutting**).

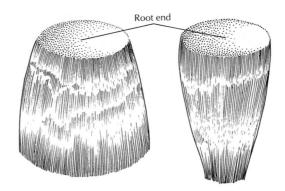

Taper cutting

Taper, **slither** or **feather** cutting will reduce both the length and the thickness of the hair. This technique is done on dry hair and, unlike club cutting, the hair is cut underneath the fingers.

Tapering is a sliding, slithering, backwards-and-forwards movement along a sub-section of hair. Close the scissor blades as you move towards the roots.

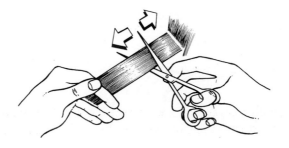

Freehand cutting

This is where the hair is cut **without being held in place** with tension from any forced directional pull. The hair is combed from its section and allowed to fall into its own natural movement before cutting.

● It is a particularly useful technique during one-length cutting, where a straight line is required. On below shoulder-length hair, holding the hair with a finger underneath can cause unwanted graduation.

● Cutting fringes with a cowlick will naturally make the hair bounce up too short if it is cut with tension.

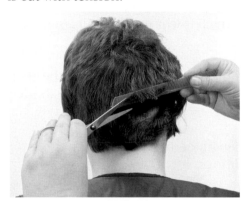
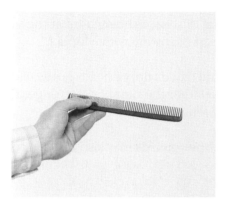

Scissor over comb

This technique is used to give the same effect as '**clipper over comb**' work. The hair around the nape and sides is cut short, following the contours of the head. Use a cutting comb to pick up the hair, keeping the scissors parallel to the comb during cutting. Use the comb in an upwards direction, lifting the hair so that the hair sticking through it can be cut off. Move the comb and scissors continually towards the top of the head, keeping the comb up and out and away from the head, cutting at the same time.

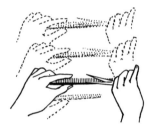

Scissor over comb

Thinning hair with thinning scissors

Thinning scissors are used for blending in weight lines and for softening hard lines, by being inserted at the ends of the hair.

These scissors remove only thickness or bulk from the hair, not length. They are sometimes called **aesculaps**, **serrated** or **texturising scissors**.

Ordinary thinning scissors can be used to thin out from the middle of the hair, cutting diagonally across the sub-section of the hair. Open and close them two or three times to remove the thickness.

Many new variations on the normal thinning scissors have now been developed, and the different shaped blades can be used to create a variety of exciting effects.

Combs

Cutting combs are normally used for cutting most hair, but thin flexible barber's combs are needed to cut around the ears and necklines for really short cuts.

TO DO

Practise holding your scissors and opening and closing the top blade with the back of your hand towards you. This is the only way you can cut the hair short enough during barbering.

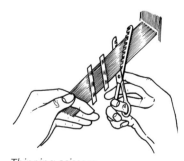

Thinning scissors

Cutting techniques using clippers and razors

Clippers

Electric clippers are now commonly used for both men's and women's hairdressing to give the same effect as the 'scissor over comb' technique.

Clippers have two blades with sharp-edged teeth. One blade remains fixed while the other moves across it. The action of the motorised moving blade is similar to several pairs of scissors being used at the same time, which is why many hairdressers like the speed of cutting with clippers.

Detachable clipper heads are available so that the closeness of the cut can be altered. The larger the number, the longer the length; the smaller the number, the shorter the length.

Clipper guards may also be used to vary the length of the cut. The sizes are:

1	or	0.15 cm ($\frac{1}{16}$ in.) (the shortest)
2	or	0.3 cm ($\frac{1}{8}$ in.)
3	or	0.6 cm ($\frac{1}{4}$ in.)
4	or	1 cm ($\frac{3}{8}$ in.) (longer hair)
		1.25 cm ($\frac{1}{2}$ in.)
		2.54 cm (1 in.)

depending on the manufacturer.

When you are cutting very short necklines clipper across the head to cross-check the cut as hair grows in all directions. If the hair grows upwards you will need to clipper the hair down in the opposite direction.

Creating patterns in the hair with clippers

Clippers are also used artistically to create patterns in the hair, known as channelling. Once a design has been agreed with the client the hairdresser can show off their creative flair and steady hand by turning the clippers face down to mark out the lines. Remember to let your client know how quickly the pattern will grow out, and to keep it fresh it will need to be done every two or three weeks. Darker hair shows the pattern better than blonde hair and patterns are best created on clean, short hair, uniformly cut 2.5 mm – 2.5 cm long.

Razors/hair shapers

These can be used to create fashion styles and are ideal for creating soft, wispy outlines and textured styles.

The two main types of razor in use are:

- Open or cut-throat razors
- Shapers or safety razors.

Both are used on wet hair because razoring on dry hair is painful for the client. Razors must be kept sharp or they will tear the hair.

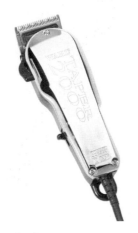
Electric clippers

REMEMBER

The bottom, static, blade of the clippers should always be further forward than the top, moving, blade. If the top blade comes too far forwards you could cut someone's skin, so be extra careful when clippers are turned over for lining out. Always put on the blade guard when clippers are not in use.

TO DO

Practise transferring designs on the head by:
- *Preparing a template, holding it against the hair and spraying*
- *Marking the design onto hair using a freehand method*
- *Using scissors to outline the design, freehand, onto the hair.*

Open or cut-throat razors

Open razors may be used to shorten the hair and to remove thickness. They are used underneath or above the wet sub-sections of hair and are stroked towards the ends with a scooping movement that produces a tapered effect. Many hairdressers also use open razors to create a clean hairline around the haircut.

It is important to hold a razor safely so that it does not close up on your hand during cutting. Open razors are now available with disposable blades. These are more hygienic, and as one blade becomes blunt you can replace it, so you always have a sharp edge to use.

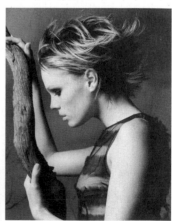

HEALTH MATTERS

Always use a new razor blade for each client if the blade is to come in contact with skin, and dispose of it in a sharps container or wrap carefully in cotton wool and paper and secure before placing in a bin.

Safety razor

Shapers or safety razors

These razors have a guard over the blade so that only part of the hair is cut. They produce a feathered, uneven effect and are easier and safer to use than open razors.

Safety razors for men's hairline shaping

Open razors with disposable blades are used for hairline shaping (lining out) and removing unwanted hair outside the desired outline shape. The best way to do this is to use a piece of cotton wool with warm water and shampoo to soften the hairs first, then stretch the skin tight before removing the hairs with the razor.

REMEMBER

Cutting to the natural hairline shape in barbering:
- Retains the neckline shape for longer
- Appears more masculine.

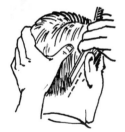

Shave outline below ear

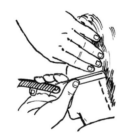

Shave left side of neck using backhand stroke

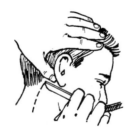

Clean neck below ear

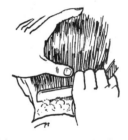

To achieve a square or precision hairstyle, shaving or precision outline is needed

REMEMBER

Always change your razor's disposable blade in front of the client so that your hygiene practices can be observed.

Combining cutting techniques

Fashion styles are created by combining a variety of basic cutting techniques to produce the desired result. Personalising the cut using texturising techniques gives an individual look.

Richard Ward

Combined cutting techniques

Texturising techniques

Listed below are some examples of texturising techniques.

Twist cutting

Twist small sections of hair and either chip into section using points of scissors or use a tapering action to remove hair.

Slicing

When the outline shape of the haircut is achieved, comb the hair into style, slightly open the blades of the scissors and position on the section of hair to be sliced, then slide blades down the section to remove hair. This technique is best used when texturising front hairlines, fringes and sides.

Pointing and texturising

Pointing can be used to achieve feathered effects and to soften hard lines created by club cutting.

Take a sub-section of hair and insert the scissors over the fingers to chip out small pieces at the ends of the hair. When larger pieces are taken out of the hair, this is called **texturising**. See colour plates 3–4.

REMEMBER

When texturising, do not use serrated-blade scissors as these will pull the hair and cause discomfort to clients.
Straight-edged blades are best.

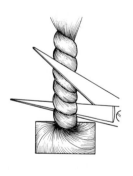

Twisting

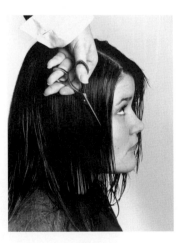

Slicing

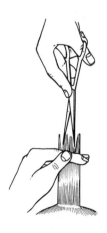

Point cutting

Weave cutting

Take a section of hair and weave, as for highlighting. Drop the hair you wish to leave longer and cut the remaining woven strands. The result can be either drastic or subtle depending on the size of the weave and the effect required. Thickly woven strands will produce a quite dramatic, severe result whilst fine strands will give a subtle result.

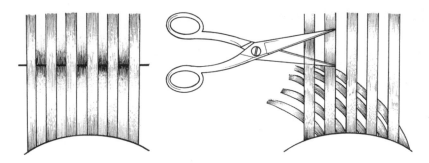

REMEMBER

It is better to take finer sections and adjust as required than risk cutting too much off.

Finishing techniques

It is important not only to have the skills to carry out cutting techniques to produce a particular haircut but also to know which products, tools, equipment and techniques can be used to dry the hair into shape and create a finished result. This will enable you to advise the client on how to recreate the style her/himself.

Cross-checking a man's haircut

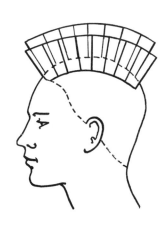

The difference between checking a man's haircut and checking a woman's haircut is that you should only cross-check a man's cut vertically. You do not cut the corners off as you would for a woman's cut. The result should be more square than round.

To check the shape and balance, look at the man's profile from all angles, not just through the mirror. Place a white towel over your shoulder (unless the hair is white, when you should use a dark towel) to give a clear background and to see the shape properly.

TO DO

Show the client how much product to use on his hair. Many clients use too much and often suffer from flaking scalps.

Once the hair is dry you can give a final shine or polish by using:

- dressing cream (which is lighter than wax) for fine light-coloured hair
- wax for darker, heavier hair.

TO DO

Find a selection of pictures that incorporate all the cutting techniques listed below and give a brief description of which cutting techniques and tools were used and what cutting angles, outline and internal shapes would be used to recreate the look. Also include details of styling and finishing techniques, products, tools and equipment used for each haircut.

- *Tapering*
- *Thinning*
- *Freehand*
- *Texturising*
- *Scissor over comb*
- *Club cutting*
- *Layering*
- *Graduation*
- *Reverse graduation.*

TEST YOUR KNOWLEDGE

1   Why should you pay attention to influencing factors when cutting hair?

2   Why should the client's lifestyle be considered when designing a hairstyle?

3   What safety considerations should you take into account when cutting hair, and why?

4   How should you dispose of hair cuttings?

5   Why is it important to consult with the client throughout the cutting process?

6   What is the best type of scissors to use when slicing the hair?

7   List the different baselines and the results produced by each.

8   List the different techniques of layering and the results produced by each.

9   When would you texturise the hair by chipping/point cutting?

10   Why is it important to ensure client satisfaction?

11   Describe what is meant by classic, fashion and emerging fashion styles.

12   Describe the differences between cutting techniques and layering techniques and how they can be used to achieve a variety of layered looks.

13   List the cutting techniques that should be used on wet hair and the ones that should be used on dry hair.

14   Why is it important to cut to the natural hairline in men's hairdressing?

15   Describe how to maintain clippers.

16   How would you prepare the hair for cutting patterns?

17   Descibe different methods of transferring designs onto the head. How would you use them?

18   Why is it important to cross-check a haircut?

19   Decribe, with the aid of sketches, the typical pattern of male baldness.

20   Why is it important to cut the natural hairline when barbering?

Chapter 4 Creative styling and extensions

Whether you are preparing a model's hair for a show, creating a style for a bride or simply adding a few neon-coloured hair extensions to add interest, having the skills and knowledge of the advanced techniques used for creating a look for a few hours or a few months takes time and practice. Many different looks can be created with a setting curler, a few pins and some added hair pieces in theatre, on television, on the catwalk and even in the salon. This chapter will help you create hair in new dimensions.

This chapter covers the following NVQ level 3 units:
H25 Style and dress hair to achieve a variety of creative looks
H26 Style and dress long hair
H23 Provide hair extension services.

Creative setting

Setting hair is not just for older clients in the salon. Many styles you see in fashion magazines and on the catwalk have been created with the help of a roller or two. Modern styles of setting can be divided into three groups:

- Classic
- Fashion
- Alternative.

Classic styles

Classic styles have timeless appeal and include dressing the hair up into **French pleats**, **chignons** and **rolls**, with longer hair being worn down in waves or smoothed under. Shorter hair can be **pin-curled** or **finger-waved** to create movement.

Fashion styles

Fashion styles are styles that are currently 'in vogue'. Setting longer hair on Molton Browners will give **spiral** or **corkscrew-type curls**, which can be separated and defined using wax. Putting in Velcro rollers using traditional methods of rollering to create volume and curl will produce soft, casual, yet fashionable styles on short, medium or long hair. Changing the **set**, or **pli**, **direction** can create many variations on one head. When putting hair up modern styling looks towards a sleeker, flatter finish with a focal point of height or volume with very little root lift in the crown area.

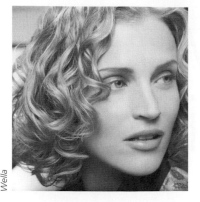

Wella

Many-strand plaits or braids can be worn up, down, or across the head and can be woven under or over to create different looks. Once the basic skills of braiding have been learned, there are many different results that can be created using variations on the same theme.

Twists, knots and rolls can all be combined to produce many fashion as well as alternative styles.

Both classic and fashion techniques of dressing hair up are very popular for special occasions such as weddings. Bridal styles often incorporate ornamentation such as fresh or synthetic flowers in the final dressing.

Alternative styles

These are the more outrageous and creative high-fashion designs, often incorporating ornamentation and added hairpieces. They are usually restricted to competition, photographic and show work. Usually the style has some basis in classic or fashion styles, but with the details exaggerated to create more dramatic results (colour plate 7).

REMEMBER

Always design the hairstyle to suit the occasion or situation for which it will be required.

REMEMBER

Setting hair with the natural fall or growth pattern will help the style to last longer. The client will also find it easier to manage.

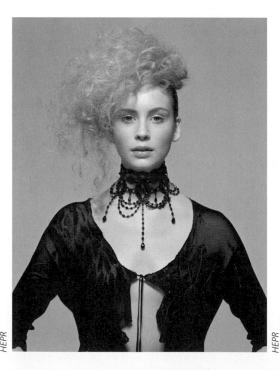

HEPR

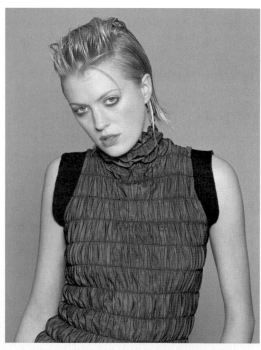

HEPR

TO DO

List the setting and dressing services offered in your salon and the time allocated for each when booking appointments.

For example, winding a spiral set using chopsticks will produce very dramatic, **tight corkscrew curls** and synthetic hair can be used when dressing hair up to give extra height and bulk, enabling very exaggerated results to be produced.

- *Using style magazines, collect examples of classic, alternative and fashion styles and consider how you would recreate each one, listing products, tools, equipment and techniques you would use.*
- *Read Chapter 1 on how to keep up to date with fashion trends.*

Client consultation

- Use your style book to discuss the style with your client and select the type of style suitable.

- Discuss the occasion with your client. Wedding or evening function?

- Discuss the clothes your client will be wearing. Do they have a high or low neckline? Will the hairstyle balance with the clothes?

- How much time will you need to dress the style? Dressing hair up will take longer.

- Discuss the cost with the client. Many salons charge extra for putting hair up.

General points to consider when deciding on a style include:

- **The shape of the head.** If it is flat at the back more hair will be needed there to balance it.

- **The shape of the face.** A round or square face can be softened by a few tendrils of hair around the face.

- **The amount of hair.** If dressing hair up, does the client have enough hair or will a hairpiece be needed?

- **Hair structure.** If the hair is very straight it will need setting first. If very curly, it may need to be straightened.

- **Hair texture.** Frizzy hair may need wax or dressing cream to smooth it. Strong, coarse hair may need a strong styling lotion for control.

- **Hair length.** The longer the hair, the heavier it becomes. This can create problems when dressing hair up.

When putting long hair up, in addition to looking at the hair we also need to consider the following:

- What is the occasion? Is the client going to a special event – ball/wedding etc.?

- What will the client be wearing? If the outfit has a low neckline, leave a few tendrils of hair hanging down – having all the hair pinned up can make the client feel bare.

- Is the outfit ornate or plain/sleek? Ornate dress with very fussy hair may look over-done – preferably keep the style simple and chic/classic. If the dress is plain then go for a more adventurous/creative hairstyle.

- Will there be a head-dress or hair ornamentation? If the headwear is very ornate, keep the style simple and uncluttered.

- Don't forget shoes – high shoes with high hairstyles could make the client look very tall (remember, the style should look balanced and in proportion).

- Does the client have a male escort/partner for the event? You will need to consider his height – creating a 'structure' that will tower over the partner will not be pleasing to the eye, or the couple concerned!

Preparation of client

Gown the client using gown and towel to protect clothing.

If the hair is being dressed up, advise the client to wear a top that does not have to be pulled off over the head as this will spoil the hairstyle – a blouse/top with buttons is best.

Consider hair preparation – does the hair need to be freshly washed? If not, ask the client to wash her hair before coming in if possible. Do you really need to set the head on traditional rollers before putting it up? This can sometimes create too much root movement (and also roller marks that are hard to disguise) – heated rollers are ideal for creating curl at the ends of the hair without too much root lift.

Bridal hair

If you do a lot of bridal hair, consider putting together a bridal package. This should include a thorough consultation, rehearsal session plus an appointment for the final date with a total price given for the package. A nice touch is to also include champagne on the morning of the wedding. For the rehearsal session you will need the head-dress and veil, and ask the client to wear something white and plain to enhance the head-dress – alternatively, keep some white and cream fabric at the salon to use. Get her to wear her wedding make-up so that a true image of the actual look can be achieved. Taking Polaroid pictures of the finished style will help when it comes to recreating the style on the wedding day and will remind the bride-to-be of what she will look like. Some salons offer make-up and manicure services; these could also be included in the bridal package.

Client satisfaction

To ensure client satisfaction, it is essential that clients are happy not only with their hairstyle but also with the hair-care advice and the general treatment they receive whilst in the salon. Before commencing any service, a thorough consultation should be carried out leading to a discussion of the style required. Combined with the practical skills of the stylist, this should ensure that clients are happy with the service they receive.

TO DO

Re-read Chapter 1 on client consultation and feedback on services provided.

Tools, equipment and products used in setting

Whether you are creating a classic, fashion or alternative style, selecting the correct tools, equipment and products is essential if the finished result is to be successfully achieved.

Brushes

These are used before setting to disentangle the hair during consultation and after setting to remove the roller marks and dress the hair.

REMEMBER

Whatever the occasion – always allocate enough time to create the look without having to rush. A practice session is a good idea as it allows you to try out a variety of different styles before the actual event and gives your client the opportunity to say how she feels – and to change her mind if necessary.

REMEMBER

The client is the most important person in the salon. If a client is not satisfied with the service they receive they will not return. A happy client will return to the salon for further treatments.

Flat brushes with open tufts or bristles are normally used as these do not get tangled in the hair.

Combs

Tail combs have plastic or metal tails and are used for sectioning the hair when inserting rollers.

Dressing-out combs can have larger teeth for disentangling hair, and fine teeth which are useful for back-combing.

Traditional rollers

These can be smooth or spiky. Spiky rollers are better for holding hair in place but can be difficult to keep clean and free from hairs, often becoming tangled in longer hair. Smooth setting rollers are more suitable for use on highly bleached or porous hair and when setting hair for competition or photographic work, as they do not leave ridges or marks on the hair.

Rollers are available in cylindrical and conical shapes.

Velcro rollers

Velcro rollers, designed for use on dry hair, have small hooks which grip the hair as it is being wound, enabling them to remain secured in the hair without the need for pins.

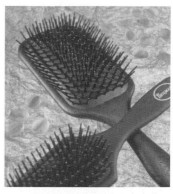
Flat/paddle brush

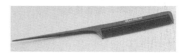
Tail comb

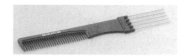
Dressing-out comb

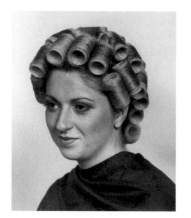

Heated rollers

These rollers are pre-heated and wound into dry hair, secured and left to cool down before removing. They are ideal for giving a quick foundation curl when putting hair up.

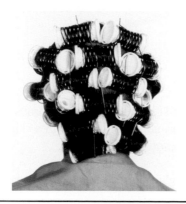

REMEMBER

Excessive use of heat and heated styling equipment can cause damage to the hair and in some cases to the scalp if care is not taken. When using heated rollers, wrap tissue paper around rollers or ends of hair before winding to diffuse heat and prevent excessive damage to hair.

Molton Browners

These come in foam or rubber and are used to give a spiral or corkscrew/ringlet effect on long hair. They will produce a curl result that is even along the hairs' length.

As with conventional setting, whichever type of curler is used, the size will determine the end result, with larger rollers producing soft results and smaller ones giving tighter curls.

Pins and clips

Straight pins are used to secure rollers during setting and for dressing long hair.

Fine hair pins are mainly used for dressing hair up and are available in several shades to match the client's hair colour.

Hair grips, like fine hair pins, are available in a variety of colours and are mostly used for long-hair dressings.

Setting nets are used to keep rollers and pin curls in place while the client is under the dryer.

Hairnets are often made from real hair and come in a variety of colours and shades. They are very useful for show or photographic work to keep long hair smooth and in place when dressing into pleats/rolls, etc., as they are extremely fine and barely visible if used correctly.

Styling and finishing products

Setting aids
Setting aids serve two main purposes: to protect the hair from the heat of the hairdryer, and to prevent the hair from absorbing moisture – which will, in turn, prolong the life of the style. They do this by coating the hair with a fine, water-soluble plastic film.

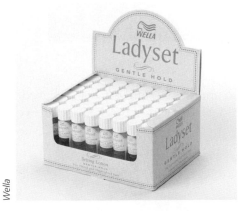

Wella

Setting lotions/gel sprays
These come in liquid form and can be runny. Gel sprays are a modern form of setting lotion and usually come in non-aerosol spray bottles. They will give a firm hold and are applied to wet hair before setting.

ADVANCED HAIRDRESSING

Mousse

Also used when wet setting, this gives a softer result than setting lotions.

Gel/sculpting lotions

These have a thicker consistency than lotions. They do not run and are ideal for sculpting or moulding the hair – for example, when creating finger waves.

Thermo-active sprays

These are used when dry-setting with Velcro or heated rollers to help hold the style. They are applied to clean, dry hair either before or after placing rollers, depending on the hair length. When setting longer hair, it is better to apply them before setting to ensure an even curl strength.

Dressing hair

Wax

This gives the longest hold and is used to prevent static, give definition and mould the hair. It can be quite heavy and can make the hair look lank and greasy if too much is applied.

Frequent use can also cause build-up.

Pomades/dressing creams

These have the same uses as wax but are lighter to use, gentler on the hair and do not leave build-up.

Shine sprays

These will give hair shine and help prevent static. They should be used sparingly as they can make the hair look greasy.

Moisturisers

Products such as Wella System Professional Active Repair fluid, often called **serums**, are moisturising products formulated for use on longer hair to smooth the hair, giving shine and accentuating the style.

Hairsprays

These are used to finish the style and to help control longer hair when dressing up.

Setting techniques

Wet setting

Setting the hair when wet will give a firmer, longer-lasting result, which is ideal when creating structured styles such as finger waves or when working on fine hair which does not hold a set well.

Dry setting

This method involves setting clean, dry hair and gives a softer, more casual result, which is ideally suited to today's fashion styles. The two most popular methods are to use Velcro rollers or heated rollers. Methods of winding are the same as when using conventional setting rollers, with the finished result being determined by the curl direction, volume created and size of rollers used.

Traditional setting methods

Traditional methods include setting on rollers, pin-curling and finger-waving. These are essential skills, learned during training, which can all be adapted and incorporated into classic, fashion and alternative hair dressings.

Alternative setting methods

Alternative setting methods include spiral winding using Molton Browners, chopsticks or rags. This method of winding is the same as when spiral winding for perm. (Chapter 6 gives a description of how to carry out the wind.)

Creative styling and finishing

Once the basic skills of setting have been mastered, the techniques can be adapted as desired to create classic, fashion or alternative styles. It is often possible to combine a variety of setting techniques – rollers, pin curls and finger waves – on one head to produce a specific 'look'.

Preparing hair for dressing out

Points to remember when dressing out:

- Remove any large earrings or necklaces that the client is wearing, in case they become entangled in the client's long hair.
- If back-combing is required, which roughens the cuticle scales to create volume, use only at the root area and not through mid-lengths and ends. When dressing the hair down, try to limit back-combing to the crown area only.
- If tying hair up in pony tails, use covered bands to prevent damage to hair.
- If using ornamentation, make sure it balances the style rather than overwhelms it.
- Hairspray – use a fast-drying hairspray with medium hold when working and switch to a stronger hold to finish.

Tip: instead of buying elastic bands, make your own using fine, rolled dressmakers' elastic – cut to size and hand knot as required.

Choosing brushes for dressing out

Smooth styles
Use an open-tufted brush such as an isnis or paddle when brushing hair out to remove roller marks. Smooth the hair into position and back-brush the crown area if required.

Curly styles
For a more casual finish, dress out the hair using your fingers or an Afro comb to separate the curls. Remember, brushing can produce a frizzy look. See colour plate 8.

REMEMBER

Allow hair to cool completely before dressing out. Taking rollers out when the hair is still warm will loosen the curl, giving a softer result.

REMEMBER

Failure to brush the hair through thoroughly before dressing it into style can cause breaks in the dressing, which are difficult to remove.

REMEMBER

Practise dressing long hair up on a practice head, or any willing clients. Good results come with practice and experience.

Dressing long hair up

Dressing longer hair up requires more practice but again, once basic styles and techniques of braiding and dressing have been achieved, it is possible to build on them and create many different results, depending on the occasion and client requirements. See colour plate 8. Hair can be manipulated into knots, rolls, twists, pleats – almost anything if you put your mind to it – and many styles can be created with one or a combination of techniques.

Curly hair – casual updo

For this style you are trying to create a casual soft shape. The 'template' is a triangular shape.

Divide hair into three sections – two front sections from a centre parting, ear to ear across crown. The whole back of the head is the third section.

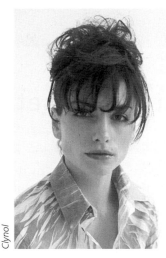

Clynol

Casual updo

Twist the back section of the hair into a loose pleat and pin, leaving curls at the crown. Twist the base of small sections of hair sticking out of pleat and grip into place to create an even shape.

For the side sections use a two-pronged setting pin in a chopstick action, swirl the hair around the ends of the pin, put into place and secure by pushing into the root area to build up the shape. Continue in this manner with all side sections until a good shape has been created. Do not use wax to finish as this can make the hair heavy, causing the style to collapse – use hairspray to give definition to the curls.

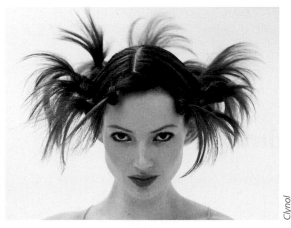

Sean Hanna

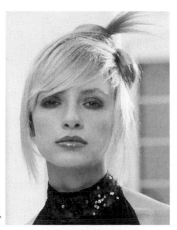

Clynol

Added hair

False hair is ideal for adding bulk and length to hair, whether dressing it up or down. This can be attached in many different ways and can be used for a couple of hours or a few months.

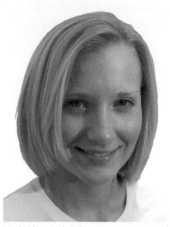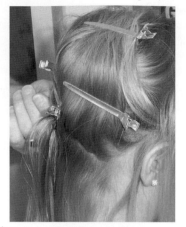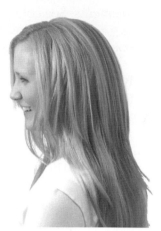

Mark Glenn Hair Enhancement www.markglenn.com

Health and safety when setting and dressing

As with any other hairdressing service, there are many health and safety considerations to be aware of. Always follow the basic rules when setting and dressing hair, including:

- Prepare all tools and equipment before use – check manufacturers' instructions if unsure.
- Ensure that you know how to use any electrical equipment, e.g. heated rollers.
- Make a visual check of electrical equipment before using to ensure it is safe to use and minimise the risk of accidents.
- Protect the client and her clothing throughout the service.
- Remember COSHH regulations – store, handle and dispose of all products used according to manufacturers' instructions and salon policy.
- Sterilise all tools and equipment before use to help prevent cross-infection.
- Maintain a professional image by keeping work areas clean and tidy.

Salon professional image

The image of the salon is portrayed through the type and standard of work (or services) it provides to its clients.

Benefits to be gained by enhancing the professional image of the salon include increased salon business, increased client take-up of new and existing salon services, greater client satisfaction and the potential to become involved with new opportunities such as hair shows, seminars, etc.

TO DO

Think of some other benefits to be gained by enhancing your salon's image and list some further ways of enhancing the image of your salon.

TEST YOUR KNOWLEDGE

1 Why is it important to consider hair fall and hair growth patterns when planning a style?

2 List the health and safety points to consider with regard to the use of equipment.

3 What are your responsibilities under COSHH regulations regarding styling and finishing products?

4 Why should you check electrical equipment before using?

5 Why is it important to avoid cross-infection and infestation?

6 Give examples of classic, fashion and alternative looks.

7 What are the best rollers to use on bleached or highly porous hair?

8 What adverse effect can excessive use of heated styling equipment have on the hair?

9 What effect will the amount of rollers used have on the finished style?

10 What effect does the size of rollers used have on the end result?

11 Give five examples of potential problems if excessive tension is used on the hair or if it is worn for a long period of time.

12 Why should you allow the hair to cool before dressing out?

13 How can humidity affect the finished style?

14 What would be the best brush to use when dressing hair into a smooth style?

15 Why should hair sections be brushed thoroughly before dressing?

16 When would you use the following products:

- Gel
- Wax
- Dressing cream
- Moisturisers
- Shine spray
- Finishing spray?

17 How can you ensure that the client is happy with the end result?

Hair extensions

The hair extension market is growing rapidly. Hair extensions, whether used for adding length, thickness or colour, can be applied in many different ways. In recent years this service has become more widely available and economical to have in the high street salon. Highly skilled professionals can create fantastic results in a few hours.

Sewing

A technique mostly used for African Caribbean hair, the natural hair is plaited into cornrows on the scalp to create a base for weave wefts to be sewn on to. The wefts are pre-made, so colour matching is very important.

Plaiting

Synthetic hair is used for this method of extensions and usually involves two people working together on four-stranded plaits. By taking very small sections of natural hair

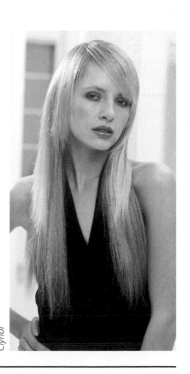

Clynol

REMEMBER

Oil sheen or serums are:
● An advantage when sewing or platting added hair
● A disadvantage when using fusing or bonding techniques.

TO DO

Use the internet or hair magazines to find different hair extension manufacturers and try to get as much information as possible on all the different techniques.

TO DO

Human hair extensions vary greatly in quality. Ask manufacturers for information on their treatment process before the hair comes to you.

TO DO

Read your salon's aftercare literature for hair extensions for clients. If your salon does not have one then write one yourself.

and dividing in two then placing a small weft of synthetic hair in the middle, the natural hair is crossed over then the synthetic hair and so on until the plait is about 1.25 cm (half an inch) long. A few strands of synthetic hair are then wrapped around the plait and fused together with special heated prongs. Skilled professionals can do this very quickly and it can be amazing to watch. Because the wefts of hair are loose, different colours can be blended to match the natural hair. Long plaits can also be created in this way with the ends of the plaits bonded to stop them unravelling.

Fusing and bonding

Fusing and bonding is a technique used for attaching small individual wefts of hair to the root of the natural hair. These extensions are almost always human hair. They come either as pre-bonded 'strands' or wefts which can be mixed for colour and bonded as they are attached. This is time consuming and can take up to four hours for one head of extensions, but the results can be dramatic.

Consultation

It is extremely important that the consultation service with hair extensions is carried out thoroughly. Some manufacturers supply forms to be filled in by the stylist during the consultation and signed by the client. This form protects the hairdresser and client from any problems which may occur due to ineffectual consultations. The hair extension service can be timely and costly so it should be given careful consideration by both hairdresser and client.

Considerations during consultation

The client's hair and scalp needs to be in reasonable condition, i.e. no signs of breakage and a normal to dry scalp (not suffering from excessive greasiness). The natural hair needs to be at least 10 cm (4 in.) long all over the head, and is always prepared by being shampooed, conditioned and dried beforehand.

Properly done, a head of hair extensions can look amazing but, of course, hair extensions are not suitable for everyone. For example, the extra weight of added hair can loosen the already weak roots of people who are having chemotherapy, or suffer from alopecia or men who are naturally losing their hair. For these people hair extensions will only quicken the inevitable hair loss.

People with skin sensitivities or a history of allergic reactions should have a 'trial run' with two or three individual extensions for a couple of weeks.

The presence of hair extensions will only aggravate skin disorders such as eczema or psoriasis and these clients should not be considered suitable for hair extensions. Because hair extensions come in different thicknesses people with very fine hair can benefit from the effect of added hair; unfortunately very sparse hair would not be suitable, as it would be difficult to disguise the attachments.

Colour mixing

Depending on the hair preparation, a mix of colours can be used so that the client can have a block colour or highlighted effect. Pre-bonded extensions and wefts of human hair can be coloured (check with the manufacturers beforehand) or a variety of coloured strands or wefts can be added to give a natural or fashion tonal look to the hair.

Loose wefts of synthetic hair can be mixed prior to application. This should be done with nimble fingers to avoid too much wastage.

The main colour should be held firmly in the palm of one hand while the secondary colour is added to the main weft in small pieces, evenly spread out and then brushed through with a soft bristle brush to mix the colours together. The more the wefts are brushed together the more blended the mix will become.

Attaching hair extensions

Every hairdresser attempting to provide hair extensions as a service to their clients should be trained by a reputable organisation. Most manufacturers provide training courses in the art of adding their hair extensions. Many factors need to be taken into account when attaching hair extensions, particularly a full head of single extensions. Look at the natural growth patterns and work with them rather than against them otherwise it will cause the client some discomfort. Look at the texture and type of the natural hair – if the hair is fine then add only fine extensions; if the hair is thick then add thicker extensions. Too much hair will cause hair breakage and scalp damage, and too little hair will not produce good results for the client. Equally, naturally curly hair should be partnered with wavy or curly hair extensions unless the client is very good at straightening their own hair to blend, but this is not recommended as stress will be put on the bindings.

When sewing or plaiting hair extensions the natural hair is completely covered or interwoven with the extensions.

HEALTH MATTERS

Traction alopecia is caused by excessive tension on the hair roots. This occurs particularly around the hairline, where the hair is naturally weaker, when the hair is pulled tight in scalp plaits or extensions over a long period of time. During consultation clients must be made aware of the problems caused by excessive tension over a long period of time. Traction alopecia is apparent when the hair becomes sparse particularly around the hairline. The hair also becomes dull, the scalp becomes sensitive and the client experiences painful raised follicles which can become infected. If there are signs of this condition the hair extensions must be removed immediately and the client should be referred to a trichologist for advice.

Cutting hair extensions

When hair extensions are added, cutting techniques need to be adapted to avoid excessive tension on the hair extensions that will cause slippage or breakage at the natural root. Texturising techniques should be use to cut the shape into the hair to avoid steps and blunt lines, which give hair extensions a 'paint brush effect'. Razors (only on wet hair) are mostly used to give a natural finish.

Sections should be drawn off the scalp to avoid getting the comb stuck in the attachments.

Finishing techniques

Human-hair extensions can be treated like the client's natural hair using hairdriers, irons, tongs, mousses and gels. Be very careful not to use too much tension when

TO DO

Look at the products used with hair extensions and read their instructions.

detangling the hair and do not use excessive amounts of serum-type products on the roots as this can cause the extensions to slip. Synthetic hair should not be subjected to any direct heat such as irons or tongs as this will melt the hair. Special products are available for synthetic and human-hair extensions, which you can get from the manufacturers.

Aftercare

All salons should have an aftercare leaflet to give the client to take home. Suitable products should be recommended. The client should be made aware of what is normal and what is not. For example:

- The first night's sleep may be a little uncomfortable because the attachments are fresh and tight. This should not carry on for a second night.
- When washing the hair extra rinsing time is necessary to remove all products as itchiness and flaking will occur if shampoo and conditioner is left on the scalp.
- Long, loose extensions should be loosely plaited at night time to avoid tangling.
- Follow the salon's recommended return visits to keep the extensions in check.
- If there are any signs of traction alopecia or excessive loss of hair extensions the client should return to the salon immediately.

REMEMBER

The scalp may be sensitive after wearing hair extensions for a while so be gentle when removing them.

Removal of extensions

Hair extensions are removed according to how they were put in.

Weaves
The cotton used for sewing in the weaves is carefully cut and the weaves removed. Then unplait the cornrows.

Plaiting
The sealed binding can be twisted to break the seal, then unravelled to expose the plait. The plait would then be undone and brushed through. For full-length plaits, use scissors to cut the band and unravel the plait.

Fusing and bonding
Special removal solution, which crystallises the bond, and a removal tool, which looks like a pair of pliers, are used to remove these extensions. Put a couple of drops of removal solution on the bond then crush with the pliers – the extension should easily slide out. If the extension does not slide out easily or at all do not force it; you will only cause the natural hair to break at the root. Use more removal solution and let it soak into the bond for a few seconds before crushing with the pliers again.

TEST YOUR KNOWLEDGE

1. Name the four types of hair extension and describe which products to use for each.
2. What are hair extensions made of?
3. Give three contraindications that would affect the application of extensions.
4. Which cutting techniques are best suited to shaping hair extensions?
5. How can different colours be added to the hair?
6. What is traction alopecia?
7. What are the timings for hair extension appointments in your salon?
8. What are the main aftercare procedures?
9. How should hair extensions be removed?

Chapter 5 Colouring

There are many reasons for a client to choose to colour their hair – to cover white hairs, enhance an existing hairstyle, or simply because they want a change of image. Before you colour a client's hair, it is important to understand the effects of colouring products on the hair, how to choose a complementary colour, how to apply a variety of colouring techniques, and what to do if a problem occurs. The colouring services offered by you and your salon should not only be for the benefit of the client but should also enhance the salon's image. It is important that hairdressers keep up to date with new techniques and methods of colouring hair so that they can provide a variety of services and satisfy the needs of each individual client.

This chapter covers the following NVQ level 3 units:
H30 Colour hair using a variety of techniques
H28 Provide colour-correction services.

Preparing the client for colouring or bleaching

Gowning up

It is best to gown up the client with a plastic or rubberised bleaching or tinting gown to protect their clothes from any chemical splashes. Most salons also use towels, shoulder capes and tissues around the neck area.

If you are using very dark colours, or the client has sensitive skin, you may also need to use protective barrier cream around the hairline.

TO DO

List the procedures for gowning and protecting clients for colouring services in your salon.

Preparation of self

Always wear gloves and apron when using colouring or lightening products, to protect your hands from chemical damage and skin irritation and your clothes from staining or damage.

Preparation of tools and equipment

Before you begin colouring, check that you have sufficient products and materials needed to carry out the technique you have chosen. Position on your trolley or work station all the tools, equipment and products necessary for you to complete the

TO DO

Briefly describe your responsibilities for dealing with stock shortages.

colouring service – this will ensure that everything is within easy reach and will help you to work more efficiently. Clean up work areas and dispose of any waste as you go along to help prevent accidents, minimise the risk of cross-infection and promote a professional image to your clients. Once you have completed your work, update any stock records to prevent stock shortages, which may cause inconvenience to clients and disruptions in salon services.

Safety points to remember

REMEMBER

If using an additional heat source bear in mind that too much heat can damage hair, particularly if using lightening products.

- Before commencing any colouring services check the manufacturer's instructions and your salon policy for the safe storage, use and disposal of colouring products.
- Carry out all necessary hair and skin tests. If colouring product is to come in contact with the client's skin, look at the manufacturer's instructions to see if they recommend carrying out a skin test before use.
- Always check the client's scalp for any inflammation, cuts or abrasions. If you are in doubt whether to proceed, ask another stylist for a second opinion.
- Clean up any spillages immediately.
- Ensure that all tools and equipment are properly sterilised by using chemicals, such as disinfectant, heat (for example an autoclave) or an ultraviolet cabinet.
- If you choose to use an additional heat source to help speed up the colouring process, make sure it is designed to be used with colouring products. Also check the equipment for electrical safety before using.
- Make sure that the client is comfortable throughout the service.
- When rinsing the hair make sure that the water temperature and flow are suitable for the client at all times. Remember – the scalp can be sensitive to water temperature after colouring.
- Staying alert to possible hazards throughout the client's visit will reduce the risk of accidents.

REMEMBER

Pre-colouring treatments may be used to even out the hair porosity by:
- Removing barriers that coat the hair by using product-removing shampoo
- Using porosity levellers
- Using restructuring treatments to strengthen the cortex.

Hair texture and porosity

Check the hair texture and porosity. Remember that some coarse-textured hair can be resistant to colour, and unevenly porous hair (dry ends) can absorb colour unevenly. Take a test cutting if you are unsure about the result.

Record cards

Quite a lot of information is needed when colouring and bleaching a client's hair, so always complete the record card straight away in case you forget any of the details. As many salons now use computers to store client information, these records are subject to regulation under the Data Protection Act 1998. Re-read the section in Chapter 1 which details the principles of this Act.

TO DO

List all of the hair and skin tests that should be carried out when colouring hair and describe why, when and how each of them should be carried out. What are the potential consequences of failing to do these tests?

TO DO

Write a list of all the colouring services provided by your salon and the time allocated for each.

Points to remember when choosing a hair colour

Client's requirements

- How light or dark (**depth**) do they want the colour?
- What **tone** do they want, e.g. red, copper, ashen?
- Use the shade chart to decide together.

Manufacturers of colouring products are regulated by the International Colour Code system (ICC), which identifies the depth and tone of colours on a colour chart.

Client's natural (base) colour

Very dark hair cannot be tinted to light blonde (you will have to pre-lighten with bleach).

Amount of white hair present

The more white hair present, the brighter any warm tones such as red and copper will show up.

Hair condition and porosity

Unevenly porous hair will absorb colours unevenly.

Hair texture and density

Some coarse-textured hair is resistant to colouring, so take a test cutting first.

Complexion and skin tones

Never colour an older client's hair too dark or too ashen – it will make them look older.

TO DO

Refresh your memory by drawing and labelling a simple diagram of a colour star/circle noting which colours neutralise unwanted tones.

REMEMBER

The true hair colur can only be seen in natural daylight. Artificial lighting may not show the true colour of the hair.

TO DO

Re-read the sections in Chapter 1 on giving advice and guidance to clients.

Bleaching hair

Hairdressers use bleach to lighten hair when other products such as highlift tints are not strong enough.

Clients who have naturally 'mousy' hair that lightens in the sunlight may wish to recreate this effect by bleaching. Blonde hair is often considered to be more flattering, especially with sun-tanned skin, and once clients have experienced being blonde they often feel that their own colour is less exciting.

Blonde highlights are easier to sell to clients, especially on layered hair where the natural-coloured regrowth is less obvious. The initial cost of highlights, especially woven highlights (which take more time) may be high, but they need to be repeated only every few months. If clients prefer a full head bleach, then the regrowth must be done every few weeks.

Bleaching materials

Emulsion bleach

Emulsion bleaches are made up of three separate parts:

- An oil or gel bleach
- Hydrogen peroxide (normally 20 vol. (6%) or 30 vol. (9%))
- Boosters or activators (sachets of powder).

From 12%	To 3%	Use 3 parts water 1 part 12%
From 12%	To 9%	Use 1 part water 3 parts 12%
From 18%	To 6%	Use 2 parts water 1 part 12%

Examples of how to dilute peroxide

Always check the manufacturer's instructions for the recommended strength of peroxide and the number of boosters or activators to use.

Make sure you mix up in the correct order. The peroxide and boosters are generally mixed first and then the oil or gel bleach is added so that it does not become lumpy. Emulsion bleaches are particularly good for whole-head and regrowth bleaches as the consistency makes them easy to apply and they are formulated to be gentle on the scalp.

TO DO

Look at the emulsion bleach left in the bowl after it has been used and see how much it has expanded due to the release of oxygen.

REMEMBER

Inhalation of powder bleach can cause damage to the mucal tissues of the mouth, nose, respiratory tract and lungs. Always mix it in a well-ventilated area.

Powder bleach

Powder bleaches are made of two parts:

- Bleach powder
- Hydrogen peroxide (normally 20 vol. (6%) or 30 vol. (9%)).

Powder bleaches have to be mixed to a smooth paste, but check the manufacturer's instructions as the amount of peroxide will vary if you are using liquid, as opposed to cream, peroxide.

Powder bleaches are also strong bleaches and are generally used for highlights and fashion effects. However, they have a tendency to dry out and become powdery if excessive heat is applied.

Always measure, check and mix bleach products carefully, checking the manufacturer's instructions. If you use peroxide that is too strong, or mixtures of bleach that are too thick, you could burn the client's scalp and give an uneven colour to the hair. Peroxide that is too weak, and bleach mixtures that are too thin, can run into the client's eyes, skin and clothes and will not lighten the hair enough.

The chemistry of bleaching

All bleaches are **alkaline** and contain **ammonia** (you can smell this quite strongly when mixing bleaches). The alkali in bleaches has two actions:

- It swells the hair and opens up the cuticle scales so that the bleach can enter the cortex and lighten the colour pigments.
- It mixes with the hydrogen peroxide and releases the oxygen, which will bleach out the colour.

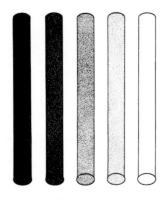

Peroxide effects

Hair when bleached will always lighten in this order:
1 Black
2 Dark brown
3 Medium red brown
4 Light warm brown
5 Light golden brown
6 Medium golden blonde
7 Light blonde
8 Very light blonde
9 White (disintegration)

Hair must **never** be allowed to lighten beyond a very light blonde colour or it will disintegrate completely.

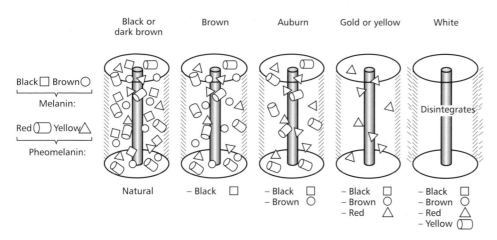

Bleaching out colour pigments

Application methods

Hair may be lightened with **highlift tint** (mixed with special developers), **emulsion bleach** or **powder bleach**, depending on the client's natural base shade and the degree of lift required. Generally, dark hair will need the stronger bleach products to lift. If in doubt, take a test cutting.

Whole head

Both whole-head and regrowth bleaches are usually applied to hair sectioned into four as shown in the diagram on the right.

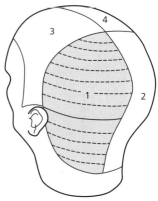

The four hair divisions

Bleach is usually applied to the nape or crown area first where the hair is more resistant. Always apply bleach to a whole head of virgin hair in this order:

1 Mid-lengths
2 Ends of the hair
3 Roots of the hair

This is because the client's body heat (from the scalp) will make the bleach take more quickly near the scalp.

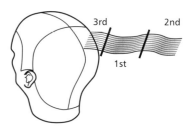

Whole head application

Never skimp with the amount of bleach. Take very small sections and always check the application thoroughly. The smallest area left uncovered will show up disastrously.

Regrowth application

When applying bleach to regrowth, always be thorough and **never overlap** on to the previously bleached hair, as hair breakage could occur.

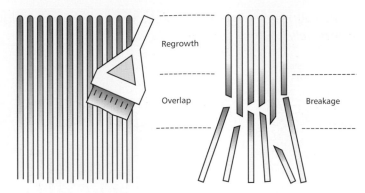

Regrowth

Overlap

Breakage

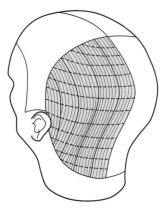

Hair breakage from overlapping

Cross-checking the application

Checking the application

You can never be too careful when applying bleach. Always check the application from the opposite direction to the one in which you applied it.

If you have missed any areas, apply bleach to them immediately, or dark patches will be seen. Pay special attention to the hairline and the thickest part of the hair (i.e. behind the ears).

Removing the bleach

Whole-head or regrowth bleach

Remove the bleach product by rinsing thoroughly until the water runs clear. Use a lower water temperature than usual because the client's scalp will be sensitive, but ask the client if the temperature is comfortable.

Then gently shampoo the hair. If a bleach toner is to be used then do not use a conditioner. Otherwise use an acid anti-oxy conditioner to return the hair to its natural pH-balanced acid state and close the cuticle scales.

Lightening and colouring products

There are many different types of colour that can be used depending on whether the client requires something long-lasting or just a temporary measure.

Temporary colours

Temporary colours are very popular because they create an instant colour change. They are quick to apply and easy to remove if the client is dissatisfied with the result.

Temporary colours are useful for adding stronger tones to natural or artificially coloured light or dark hair, e.g. warm golden, ashen, rich auburn.

Sometimes natural white hair or bleached hair looks too yellow or golden (brassy) and benefits from being neutralised by silver tones.

However, blending in a few grey hairs may be more difficult – remember that grey hair consists of white and naturally coloured hair mixed together. Some colours produce unwanted warm (orange/red) overtones on white hair.

Temporary colours can also be used to darken natural and artificially coloured hair.

The chemistry of temporary colours

The pigment molecules of temporary colours are too large to enter the hair shaft, so they coat the outside of the hair. This is why they are washed away so easily.

However, unevenly porous hair (e.g. permed and highlighted ends) will always take a temporary colour unevenly. The cuticle scales are swollen and open in porous hair and the large colour molecules can become trapped and not wash out.

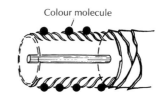

The chemistry of temporary colours

Semi-permanent colours

Semi-permanent colours have the advantage of colouring and conditioning hair at the same time. They do not need to be mixed with hydrogen peroxide and so do not leave any regrowth.

They are useful for blending in a small amount of white (grey) hair, but are not strong enough colours to cover a lot of white hair.

The chemistry of semi-permanent colours

The pigment molecules of semi-permanent colours are smaller than those of temporary colours and so are able to penetrate a little way into the cortex of the hair. They tend to wash out slowly and so last longer than temporary colours.

Unevenly porous hair (e.g. permed, relaxed or bleached hair) will also take a semi-permanent colour unevenly. The cuticle scales are swollen and open in porous hair and the smaller molecules can penetrate deeper into the cortex in the porous part of the hair, although they rinse off normally from the non-porous parts – producing patchy results.

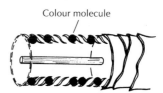

The chemistry of semi-permanent colours

Quasi-permanent colours

Some of the newer semi-permanents now last up to 15 shampoos because they contain a stronger ingredient called **para**. For these, the client must have a skin test. These colours are different because they are always mixed with a low strength of hydrogen peroxide and are known as **quasi-**, or sometimes **oxy-permanents**. They give a better coverage of white hair and an excellent shine, but can leave a slight regrowth.

Permanent colours

There are three main types of permanent hair colour.

Natural vegetable dyes

The most common of these is **henna**, which gives copper or red tones to the hair. It works by coating the hair shaft and sticking to the outside cuticle layer.

Metallic dyes

These are sold in shops as hair **colour restorers** (e.g. Grecian 2000). Never perm, tint or bleach over hair coloured using metallic dyes as it can break off as a result of the hydrogen peroxide in tint, bleach or neutralisers reacting with the metal salts deposited within the hair by the metallic dye.

Synthetic dyes

Permanent tints are para dyes and are known as oxidation dyes because they are always mixed with hydrogen peroxide.

TO DO
Re-read the section in Chapter 1 on incompatibility tests (page 23).

The widest possible choice of colours is available with permanent tints. They can be used to darken or lighten (up to four shades lighter), and have a whole range of subtle and vibrant tones.

Forms of tint available

Creams (tube)
These are mixed to a creamy consistency and are particularly good for covering coarse, resistant hair.

Oil-based tints (bottle)
These liquids mix to a gel-like thickness and give a more natural finished look.

Oil/cream emulsion (tube/bottle)
These have the benefits of both creams and gel tints and are easy to work with.

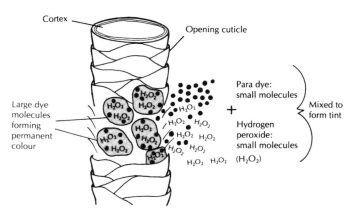

The chemistry of permanent colours

THE pH VALUE OF PRODUCTS	
Stabilised hydrogen peroxide	4
Temporary colour	4–5
Semi-permanent colours	8
Quasi- and permanent colours	9
Bleach	8–9.5

The chemistry of permanent tints

Tints are alkaline so will swell the hair and open up the cuticle scales, allowing the colour to enter the cortex.

All tints are made of small molecules of para dye mixed with hydrogen peroxide. These small molecules of tint link with the hydrogen peroxide inside the hair shaft to form larger molecules which cannot escape. This is called an **oxidation reaction**.

Once the colour has developed it remains permanently inside the hair shaft, and a pH-balanced **acid anti-oxy rinse** is applied after shampooing to close down the cuticle scales.

TO DO

Contact various manufacturers' representatives and technicians to discuss the range of colouring products they offer.

Conventional colouring and bleaching techniques

The following techniques can be carried out on a daily basis in the salon and used to create commercial results.

Woven highlights and lowlights

These are done with foil, 'Easi-Meche' or colour wraps – or, if lowlighting only, a spatula (made by Wella) can be used. Preparing woven highlights is a highly skilled technique.

Prepare the hair by sectioning in the 'nine-section' method so that you can work methodically, step by step. Take sub-sections of hair of a similar size to those used for perming, and weave out the hair with a pin-tail comb. Place the woven strands onto the correct length of foil or Easi-Meche, apply bleach, then re-seal the packets. Always start from the nape and work upwards.

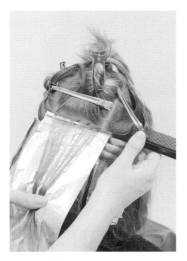
Weave hair

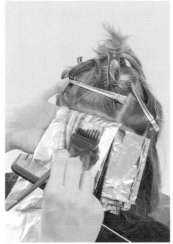
Apply product

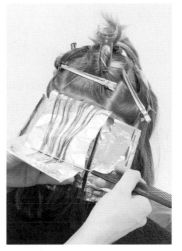
Fold foil lengthways

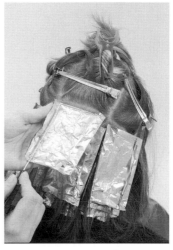
Complete parcel

When weaving out the strands of hair, always check that the strand directly below is woven, or the client will end up with stripes. As this is a lengthy process, some of the highlights may develop to the required degree of lightness before completion, so check the development continually. If some highlights are ready, then stop the development on those strands only with cotton wool and warm water. Remember not to disturb the packets still in place otherwise seepage and leaks may occur.

You might have to re-mix some fresh bleach if it takes you a long time (i.e. over 45 minutes) to complete the head, as the bleach mixture loses its strength after a time.

The advantage of woven highlights is that they are more comfortable for the client. They also allow you to see exactly where the highlights are being placed, and to mix tint and bleach highlights. The product can also be applied closer to the root area than with the cap method.

TO DO

Practise woven highlights on models who can spare the time, using thick conditioning cream instead of bleach.

REMEMBER

Always protect your skin by wearing gloves when applying bleach or colour.

REMEMBER

It is important to consider the image of the client when colouring hair. You need to ensure that the new colour will complement and enhance the personality and appearance of the client and also suit her/his lifestyle.

Lowlights

Lowlights are colours which are darker or have more tone than the client's natural base shade (e.g. golden, warm, red or silver). These are applied in the same way as woven highlights. Often two or three colours are used together for woven highlights to give many varied and natural effects. For instance, gold, copper, and light red colours woven alternately on to a dark blonde base can look particularly good.

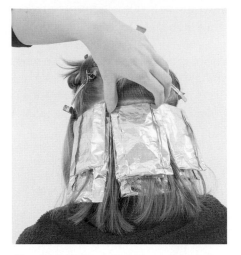
Bleach highlights with foil

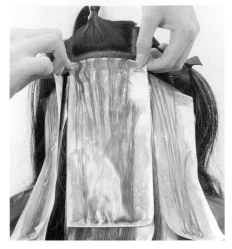
Tint lowlights with adhesive strips

Whole-head tint application

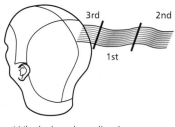
Whole-head application

For a whole-head application the tint is always applied to the mid-lengths and ends, then to the roots of the hair, unless the hair is very short. This is because heat from the client's scalp makes the tint take more quickly on the roots, which speeds up the processing time. Apply tint to mid-lengths and ends of hair and leave to develop for half the development time. Mix up fresh tint and apply to the root area, develop for a further 30 minutes and then remove. This method is used when lightening or using red/copper shades. When tinting hair darker, the colour can be applied from roots to ends in one application.

Developing and timing the tint

- Make sure that the hair is sufficiently loosened to allow the circulation of air.
- Check the manufacturer's instructions to see how long it should be left before checking (the average time is 30 minutes), and whether you should use heat (from an accelerator), which will halve the development time.
- Check the colour development by taking a strand test. Remove some of the colour from the roots and the ends and compare the two colours. If they are of the required shade, then remove the colour.

Removing the tint

Take the client to the wash-basin and add a small amount of water to loosen the colour whilst massaging the head. Rinse off the tint thoroughly with tepid water until the water runs clear. Using a cream or an acid-balanced shampoo, massage gently, then rinse. Apply a second shampoo if necessary.

Use a pH-balanced acid anti-oxy conditioning rinse to prevent the tint from oxidising any further and to close the cuticle scales. Complete the record card.

Alternative techniques

These can be used to enhance fashion styles for more adventurous clients and adapted to produce a variety of results.

Random highlights

For a step-by-step explanation of the technique used to create this effect see colour plate 6.

Tipping

This creates blond/lighter effects on the tips of the hair to emphasise the shape of the haircut.

This technique can be combined with full-head colouring on short hair. After applying tint, prepare hair as above and process, while tint is still on hair.

When lift is achieved, rinse out bleach and emulsify the tint through to the ends of the hair for 5–10 minutes. This will give the hair the same tone but lighter depth than the roots.

Method
Take triangular sections of hair, pull into an upright position and wrap foil around mid-lengths and roots to make the hair stand on end. When all areas to be coloured are prepared in the same way, apply bleach or lightening tint to the hair ends and process until desired degree of lift is achieved.

Scrunch colouring
This technique is best suited to curly styles.

Method
- Dry the hair in the desired style
- Mix colouring/lightening product
- Put on plastic/rubber gloves and paint colour onto palms and fingers
- 'Scrunch' the colour onto the hair
- Repeat the process until all areas are coated with colour. Leave to process until the desired shade is achieved, then remove the colour.

Block colouring

This involves colouring or bleaching sections of hair to create a contrast. The size of the sections taken will depend on the hairstyle and desired result. Thin sections will give a subtle effect, thicker sections will give a bolder, more dramatic result. See colour plate 7.

Method
- Once you have decided on the areas of hair to be coloured, section the hair as appropriate, ensuring that any hair not to be coloured is clipped out of the way.

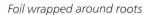

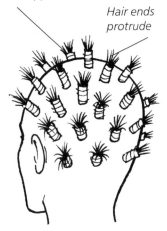

Foil wrapped around roots
Hair ends protrude

Tipping

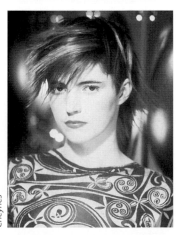

REMEMBER
Highlift tints or bleach will give best results.

Cheynes

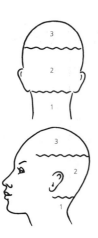

Tier colouring and sectioning

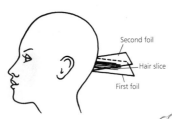

Back-to-back slices

- If colouring a small amount of hair, place a strip of foil under the section, apply colour or bleach and fold foil as for foil highlighting, to cover the hair. Leave to process and remove as per manufacturers' instructions.
- If colouring a large block of hair, after sectioning, apply colouring product to the whole section as if colouring a full head.

Graduated/tier colouring

This technique is carried out using three different colours, starting with a darker colour in the nape area and grading to lighter shades throughout the mid and top areas of the head. The technique is best suited to graduated hairstyles which are cut shorter into the nape.

Method
Divide the head into three separate areas using zigzag sections. Apply the darkest colour to the nape area. Once this is completed apply the mid-shade to the central section. Finally, apply the lightest shade to the top area and process as normal.

Back-to-back slices

This technique can create dramatic results on medium to long layered styles and is best used on the top section of the hair. It can be carried out using a variety of colours depending on client requirements.

Method
Take a section through the top of the head no longer than the width of a foil strip. Starting on the front hairline weave and wrap the section as for foil highlights. For the next section, take a fine slice of hair, place foil underneath and paint on colour, then place another piece of foil directly on top of the colour. Take the next slice of hair and lay it onto foil, apply colour and place foil on top (like a sandwich with the hair as the filling) – alternate colours should be used for best results. Continue in this manner throughout the top section of the hair.

Tip: To prevent foil slipping, slide your tail comb along the foil to make it stick to the hair beneath.

TO DO

- *Think of ways you could enhance the hairstyles of your existing clientele through the use of conventional or fashion colouring techniques.*
- *Make a list of the tools and equipment you could use to carry out the techniques listed above.*

Colour correction

There are many categories of colour correction, from simple examples such as colour fade, seepage of lightening products when highlighting or hair which has become highly lightened by the sun, to the more complex types of colour correction and colour removal techniques. Colour removal can be used for a variety of reasons, from removing tone or green discoloration from the hair to removing a build-up of dark colour. Colour removal can be used to remove semi-permanent, quasi- and permanent colours from hair. Reasons for carrying out colour removal include unsuccessful results when hair is tinted, the client wanting to change his or her hair colour, or even to recolour hair after a competition.

In some cases total colour removal is necessary, in others the hair may need to be lightened by only a few shades to remove depth or the intensity of red/copper tones. Before attempting any type of colour correction, consider the following points:

- Don't promise anything to the client – analyse the hair and give realistic advice as to what can be achieved.
- Whatever you decide to do, keep it simple and commercial – it may be easier to restyle the hair than to carry out expensive treatments that may need to be repeated frequently.
- If you do decide to go ahead with major colour removal or correction work, prepare your client – advise of the likely duration and costs of the service(s) being carried out, and whether they will need repeat appointments.
- Let the client know of any drastic changes to expect – e.g. going from blonde to red before arriving at the target shade – this will help prevent shocks later.
- Finally, make sure that you get a level of commitment from the client – you need to know that, if a series of expensive treatments is required, the client will be committed to seeing them through.

During consultation gain as much information about the hair as possible. If in doubt carry out a test cutting and assess results. Once you begin your service talk the client through what you are doing, reassess the hair at each stage and keep checking stages after application – your options could change as the work progresses.

Once colour correction work is complete always recommend aftercare products and services in order to maintain the finished result.

Types of colour removal product

Colour reducers

Sometimes called **colour strippers**, these remove artificial colour pigment only, these are hydrogen based and work by breaking down the large colour molecules into smaller ones which are easily washed from the hair.

TO DO

When carrying out colour corrections, sometimes you will need help from another member of staff. Read chapter 10, page 206 about training and development.

REMEMBER

Plan your time effectively. Look at salon time available and, where possible, try to book the appointment on a different day to the consultation as this will allow you to allocate enough time to do the job and give you time to prepare. It also gives the client a chance to prepare for the changes that will take place.

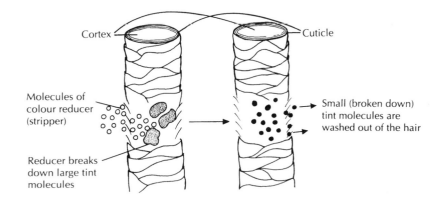

Cortex

Cuticle

Molecules of colour reducer (stripper)

Small (broken down) tint molecules are washed out of the hair

Reducer breaks down large tint molecules

The chemistry of colour strippers

TO DO

Read manufacturers' instructions on how to use colour reducers.

Bleach or oxidation-type products

These are bleaching agents that work in the same way as most bleaches, and remove natural colour pigment as well as artificial colour pigment.

Contraindications to colour removal

The following circumstances would prevent colour removal taking place:

- Presence of contagious or infectious conditions of the hair and scalp.
- Hair that has poor elasticity or is highly porous.
- Incompatible chemicals have been used on the hair, for example products containing metallic salts.
- A client shows a positive reaction to a skin test.
- A poor colour result on a strand test.
- A client with a very sensitive scalp.
- A build-up of dark products on the hair, which would be difficult to remove.

Before starting:

- Carry out a thorough client consultation, including colour analysis, and ensure that the client is happy with the chosen colour.
- Make sure that the hair is in good condition before starting.
- Always carry out appropriate tests – porosity, elasticity, skin, incompatibility and strand tests – and ensure results are satisfactory before colour removal.
- Make sure that both you and the client are well protected.

During the process:

- Do not allow any metallic objects to come in contact with the products being used.
- Always work methodically and quickly.
- Never allow the product to come into contact with any hair not being treated. When de-colouring specific areas, block off any hair not to be treated.
- Check application thoroughly.
- Avoid the use of a steamer for processing as this could cause the product to become diluted or run onto hair not being treated.
- Treat the hair and scalp gently when removing product.
- Pay attention to Health and Safety and COSHH regulations regarding yourself and your client at all times.
- Always give aftercare advice. Remember, the client's hair is now highly processed and must be treated with care.

Lightening artificial colour

To remove unwanted tone

This method will not lighten hair colour but removes unwanted tone – for example, ash tones, chlorine green or build up of temporary colour.

Method

Mix one scoop of powder bleach with 60 ml warm water. Pre-shampoo and towel dry the hair, then apply the mixture to the hair using a sponge. Develop visually by watching until unwanted tone is removed. Once the desired amount of colour has been removed shampoo and condition hair.

To remove depth and tone
A cleansing shampoo, or bleach bath, can be used to remove depth and tone and is particularly good for removing red tones.

Method
Mix one scoop powder bleach with 60 ml warm water, 15 ml shampoo and 30 ml 6% hydrogen peroxide. Pre-shampoo and towel dry the hair then apply the mixture to the hair using a sponge (remember this mixture is quite runny) on the areas needing colour removal. Visually develop as before – look for the shade of lift required. If the desired lift is not achieved after 30 minutes, remove and re-apply (you can reduce the amount of water to 30/40 ml for the second application). Rinse off and assess result – if happy, shampoo and condition hair as normal.

To remove maximum depth and tone
Full-strength bleach can be applied to the hair – but this can be used only if the hair condition is very good and test cuttings show a positive colour result.

Pre-pigmentation

This is a technique used to replace yellow, orange or red pigments into bleached hair before tinting the hair back to its natural base. If this is not done, the resulting colour will be green or ashen.

When carrying out pre-pigmentation, always refer to the manufacturer's instructions for the most suitable method of application, as this can vary from product to product. Below are two examples of pre-pigmenting techniques.

Methods
1 Apply a yellow, orange or red-toned semi-permanent to the hair and develop. Blot off excess colour with cotton wool. Apply chosen permanent colour and process as normal.
2 Use a permanent colour with a strong yellow, orange or red tone mixed with water. Apply to dry hair, blot off excess product and apply the chosen target shade.

Pre-softening

This is carried out before tinting very resistant hair to ensure good coverage and a satisfactory end result.

Method
Apply 20 vol. (9%) hydrogen peroxide to the resistant areas using a tinting brush or cotton wool. Place the client under a pre-heated hood dryer, or accelerator, until the hair is dry, then proceed with the tint application as normal.
Tip: Cream peroxide is easier to use and control than liquid peroxide.

REMEMBER
You may need to pre-pigment the hair before re-colouring with target shade.

REMEMBER
When using a bleach-type product, do not apply to root area if regrowth is present – it will bleach the natural colour.

REMEMBER
The pre-pigment colour chosen will depend on how dark or light the target colour is. Light bases will need a yellow tone, medium shades a copper tone and dark shades will need a red tone.

REMEMBER
Always use a base shade one shade lighter than required as porous hair will produce a darker result.

REMEMBER
As when pre-pigmenting, always check the manufacturer's instructions for the best possible method of pre-softening.

Counteracting colour fade

There are many causes of colour fade. These include porosity of hair and the effects of sun and sea. The method used to counteract colour fade will depend on the amount of fade that has taken place.

Minimum fade

This is when the hair has lost tone only. The technique used is often called a 'comb through' and can be carried out in a variety of ways, one example of which is given here.

Method
Apply tint to root area as normal. Once this colour has developed sufficiently, dampen the ends of the hair using water and massage the tint through from the roots to the ends of the hair. As the tint is alkaline and will cause the cuticle, or outer layer, of the hair to swell and open, it is advisable not to comb the hair too much at this stage. A good tip is to use the back of a wide-toothed comb to spread the colour and avoid damaging the hair. Once the tint is evenly distributed, leave to process for 5–10 minutes, carry out a strand test to assess results and then remove the tint as per the manufacturer's instructions.

Medium fade

In this instance the hair has lost depth of colour as well as tone.

Method
Mix tint and apply to root area as normal. Immediately you have done this, mix up a colour rinse consisting of 60 ml warm water, 15 ml 9% (20 vol.) hydrogen peroxide and 15–30 ml of tint; the amount of tint used will depend on the shade of colour being used – for strong red or copper shades use more tint in the mixture. This formula can be mixed in a bowl and applied with a tint brush or an applicator flask. Apply product straight through mid-lengths and ends of the hair and leave to develop for 30 minutes. Carry out a strand test after developing to assess results then remove product, shampoo and condition the hair as usual.

Maximum fade

For extreme loss of depth and tone an **anti-fade colour bath** is required. This process involves two stages.

Stage 1
As for previous processes, apply tint to root area. Immediately mix 45 ml of warm water with 15 ml of tint and apply to the mid-lengths and ends of the hair; again, if using a strong red shade the mixture can be altered to 30 ml tint and 30 ml warm water. Develop for 30 minutes.

Stage 2
Stabilise the colour by using a mixture of 40 ml warm water and 10 ml 9% hydrogen peroxide to expand the colour molecules, thus making the colour permanent. Pour the mixture through mid-lengths and ends of the hair and work it in with the fingers. Leave for five minutes to develop, rinse to remove and shampoo and condition the hair as normal.

REMEMBER

If the client has an ash-toned colour, substitute this with a natural shade for the colour bath as the hair can be left with a grey/green cast.

COLOURING AND BLEACHING FAULTS AND CORRECTIONS

Fault	Causes	Correction
Hair damage/breakage	Applying bleach (overlapping) onto previously bleached hair. Incorrect proportions of mixture or too many boosters/activators used. Too high a concentration of hydrogen peroxide used. Over-developing the bleach, leaving it on too long (often due to not taking a strand test). Processing with too much heat	Re-condition the hair and apply restructurants
Skin/scalp damage	Not using barrier cream around the hairline. Use of too strong a bleach mixture. Over-developing the bleach: leaving it on too long. Cuts and abrasions on the scalp before bleaching	If just a little sore, then apply a moisturising cream. If very inflamed, seek medical attention
Hair not light enough	Client's base colour too dark for the strength of bleach mixture used. Bleach mixture too weak: peroxide strength too low. Insufficient development time: bleach not left on long enough	Test hair elasticity and porosity: if satisfactory then re-bleach. Apply a silver, ash or matt toner (for yellow, orange or red hair tones)
Hair over-lightened	Use of too strong a bleach mixture. Over-developing the bleach: leaving it on too long	Re-condition the hair, apply restructurants. Re-colour under supervision
Uneven bleaching result	Uneven application. Overlapping. No allowance made for body heat on a whole-head application. Bleach mixed badly, lumps left in the mixture. Sections too large. Application too slow	Spot-bleach darker areas and re-bleach if under-processed
Hair accepts pre-pigment colour but not target shade	Hair may be overprocessed	Re-colour using half base shade + half target shade
Colour result does not match target shade	Colour under-processed (not timed accurately). Wrong strength of peroxide used. Wrong colour chosen. Client's natural base too dark for colour chosen	Re-tint hair

Cont.

COLOURING AND BLEACHING FAULTS AND CORRECTIONS (CONT.)

Fault	Causes	Correction
Patches of colour at root area after highlighting	Colour has seeped during bleaching	Spot-colour using tint to match natural base
Result too yellow after bleaching	Bleach underprocessed/too weak peroxide strength used	Re-apply bleach and process until desired result is achieved
Uneven result when tinting	Uneven application. Sections too wide. Colour mixed incorrectly	Spot-colour areas that have been missed
Skin staining	Poor application of product. Barrier cream not used before applying colour	Use stain-removal product

TO DO

Check the manufacturers' instructions of the tinting products you use for their guidelines on dealing with colour fade.

TO DO

List the limits of your authority when dealing with problems when colouring and who you would refer a problem to if you could not deal with it yourself.

TEST YOUR KNOWLEDGE

1 Draw and label the colour star and relate it to the principles of colour correction.
2 Describe how natural and artificial light affect the appearance of hair colour.
3 Why is it important to carry out hair and skin tests before and during colouring processes?
4 What personal protective equipment should be used when colouring, and why?
5 How should you dispose of any unused colouring products?
6 Why is it important to notify stock shortages?
7 List three methods of sterilising that can be used.
8 Why is it important to position equipment for ease of use?
9 Why is it important not to inhale powder bleach?
10 Why should you consider the image of the client when colouring hair?
11 Why is it important to consider the image of the salon when carrying out colour work?
12 When would you use pre-pigmentation?
13 Why would you pre-soften hair?
14 How would you dilute 12% hydrogen peroxide to form 3% and 9%; how would you dilute 18% hydrogen peroxide to form 6%?
15 Give reasons for carrying out a colour removal or correction.
16 Give the pH value of hydrogen peroxide; bleach; temporary, semi-permanent, quasi-permanent and permanent colours.
17 List the common colouring faults and how to correct them.
18 List and describe the range of colouring and lightening products available for use.

Chapter 6 Perming

The word perm conjures up all sorts of terrible images of frizzy hair and bubble looks. This is not the case for modern perming now, which is more often referred to as 'movement' or 'style support', as this is the role most perms have in hairdressing today. If you want to provide perming as a service in the salon, learning new techniques, using new equipment and products, which will please your clients and win their custom, is very important. Fantastic results can be achieved with a little imagination and expertise.

This chapter covers the following NVQ level 3 unit:
H29 Perm hair using a variety of techniques.

Client consultation for perming

A good perm depends not only on your practical skills but also on your ability to make the right decisions about your client's hair, both before and during perming. Prior to perming, carry out a thorough hair and scalp analysis, ensuring that there are no contraindications, for example infectious or contagious conditions, scalp abrasions or non-contagious disorders such as psoriasis. Make sure that the hair is in good enough condition to withstand a perm. Listed below are some points to help you when carrying out a consultation.

TO DO

Write a list of all the perming services provided by your salon and the time allocated for each.

Cutting

Most hair will need cutting, either to remove any perm on the ends or to re-style before perming. Some hairdressers prefer to cut the hair before perming, others choose to cut after perming.

When using a perm for more creative effects or adding body and volume to the hair, it is advisable to cut the hair into style before you begin your wind, as this will allow you to see exactly where lift, texture and movement are needed within the hairstyle.

REMEMBER

Small cuts or abrasions on the scalp can be protected using Vaseline or barrier cream.

Finishing techniques

During consultation the stylist must establish how much time the client will spend on the upkeep of their new style and also how they will look after their new perm. Remember – soft, big curls, waves and volume will not last as long as a traditional perm and the client must be advised of this. Very often a client will have a picture showing the look they wish to achieve, and in some cases the hair in these pictures has been styled after perming by setting or tonging. As hairdressers we must explain to the client what they would/will have to do to recreate the look they want or we have created

TO DO

Look through some style magazines and consider the products, tools and equipment that would be needed in order to recreate various styles.

for them. Take time during the consultation process to explain how the client can maintain their style at home using suitable shampoos and conditioners, styling and finishing products, tools and equipment.

Perming tests

It is important to carry out diagnostic tests both **before** and **during** the perming process. This will help to ensure that the correct products, tools, equipment and winding techniques are used. It also minimises the possibility of any problems arising and ensures the best possible results.

> **TO DO**
>
> Re-read the sections in Chapter 1 on the following tests that are relevant to perming:
> - Elasticity tests
> - Porosity tests
> - Incompatibility tests
> - Development test curls.
>
> Note the purpose of each test and the method of carrying it out.

Perming coloured and bleached hair

Hair that has been permanently coloured or bleached is more porous and will absorb perm lotion very quickly. You must, therefore, choose a strength of lotion especially for this type of hair (often no. 2, 3 or 4 strength; you will need to refer to the manufacturer's instructions).

Some hair is unevenly porous (e.g. very dry ends) and will need a **pre-perm lotion** applied to those areas of hair to even out the porosity. Pre-perm lotions are applied to towel-dried hair and left on; they are not rinsed out before perming. Pre-perm lotions usually come in liquid form and have three functions:

- They even out the porosity of the hair, thus allowing the perm lotion to penetrate the hair evenly and process all parts of the hair at the same rate.
- They maintain the hair's natural moisture level throughout the perming process.
- They help to keep the hair damp, reducing the need to keep spraying the hair with water.

Some products also contain agents that can protect the client's scalp, preventing scalp irritation.

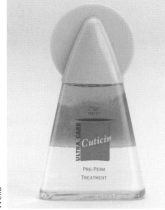

Some companies also produce **perm regulators**. This type of product usually comes in the form of a thick gel and is designed for use when carrying out any type of wind where some sections of hair do not require perming or on hair which may already have curl in the mid-lengths and ends and is in need of re-perming at the root area only. They work by restricting the amount of lotion that enters the cortex of the hair that the perm regulator has been applied to, allowing a small amount of lotion to penetrate but not enough to break any bonds.

During the consultation process the client responses to questions should be recorded then signed by the client to safeguard from any possible legal disputes.

Many salons use special consultation sheets for this purpose.

The chemical process of perming

Understanding the chemical process of perming will help you to select the correct type of lotion for your client's hair.

There are three stages in perming:
1 **Softening** – the hair is softened by the perm lotion
2 **Moulding** – the lotion causes the hair to take up its new shape whilst it is wound around the perm rods
3 **Fixing** – the hair is fixed permanently using neutraliser.

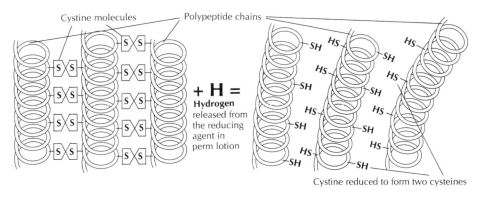

Breaking the disulphide bonds   *Hair moulded into shape around the perm rod*

Softening and moulding the hair during perming

The strong disulphide bonds in the hair are made of an amino acid called **cystine**. These are the bonds that are broken by the perm lotion during the perming process. These bonds are broken because alkaline perm lotions contain a reducing agent called **ammonium thioglycollate** (you can smell the ammonia when you open the bottle).

Most perms will process without the use of additional heat. However, if the salon is cold, the processing time can be speeded up by using an additional heat source such as an **accelerator**. Always check the manufacturer's instructions to see if they recommend using additional heat.

REMEMBER

An 'S'-shaped curl movement should be formed when the processing stage of an alkaline perm is complete, and the hair will separate into strands on an acid perm. If you see a definite 'S' formation on an acid perm this shows that the hair is overprocessed.

REMEMBER

Always read your manufacturers' instructions relating to the mixing, application and timing of perm lotions and neutralisers before using.

When using perm lotion and neutraliser accurate timing and thorough rinsing are essential to ensure best results – that enough sulphur bonds are broken and reformed to ensure that the new shape is fixed, and to prevent hair damage or deterioration of hair condition.

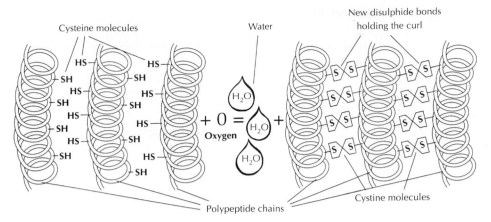

Cysteine molecules

Water

New disulphide bonds holding the curl

H_2O

$+ O =$ Oxygen

H_2O

$+$

H_2O

Polypeptide chains

Cystine molecules

Disulphide bonds broken by perm lotion   *Hair fixed in its new curled shape*

As the perm lotion soaks through the cuticle scales and enters the cortex, the reducing agent adds hydrogen to the disulphide bonds, to form a new amino acid, **cysteine**. The hair is now softened and will mould itself to the shape of the perm rods. Once the correct degree of curl is achieved neutralising agents containing either hydrogen peroxide or sodium bromate, which produce oxygen, are applied to the rods in order to fix the hair into its new position.

Neutralisers come in a variety of forms and concentrations. Some can be applied directly to the perm rods from an applicator bottle; others require dilution before application by sponge or in an applicator flask. Most neutralisers require a development period, but some now work instantly on contact with the hair. These products are often more beneficial when neutralising fashion winds.

Conditioning the hair after perming

Once neutralising is complete, applying an **anti-oxidant conditioner** to the hair will replace moisture, close the cuticle, restore the hair to its natural pH level and prevent any neutraliser that may remain in the hair from continuing to oxidise (sometimes known as **creeping oxidation**).

HEALTH MATTERS

Perming

Always remember health and safety when perming. If using cotton wool around the hairline, dampen with water first. Never leave sodden cotton wool in contact with the client's skin – remove and replace with fresh cotton wool frequently. Only apply perm lotion to the rods and never flood the scalp with lotion as this could cause skin irritation or scalp burns.

Choosing an acid or an alkaline perm

Alkaline perms

These have a pH of approximately 9.5, which opens up the cuticle scales, makes the hair more porous, and allows the perm lotion to enter the cortex.

The higher the perm lotion's pH, the more damaging it is to the hair. This is why conditioning agents are added to alkaline perms, and why acid perms are becoming increasingly popular.

Acid perms

These have **activators** added to them and generally rely on heat to open up the cuticle scales so that they can penetrate the cortex. The exception to this is when using an acid perm on bleached hair: as the cuticle layer is already damaged, additional heat may not be necessary. Remember: always check the manufacturer's instructions as products will vary. They generally have a slightly acid pH (5.5–7) and contain a chemical called **glyceryl monothioglycollate**.

Fewer bonds in the hair are broken by acid perms, which is why they are said to be better for use on damaged hair and hair that is easy to process.

Matching hair type to perm lotion

The choice of lotion type and strength is dependent upon the hair and scalp analysis and test results. Perm lotions are available for many different types of hair:

- **Resistant** – non-porous, fine hair which often dries very quickly, or some types of coarse white hair
- **Normal** – virgin hair that has not been treated with chemicals
- **Tinted** – hair that has been processed with permanent tints
- **Bleached** – hair that has been processed with bleach (including highlights)
- **Over-porous** – hair that is in a very dry, porous condition.

Hair that is generally more porous needs a weaker perm lotion, and resistant hair needs a stronger perm lotion. **But whatever type of lotion is used, always adhere to the manufacturer's instructions on suitability and use.**

After using products and materials for perming, always update stock records and report any stock shortages to the relevant person for action. Shortages of stock can lead to inability to carry out some perming services.

REMEMBER

Acid perms must be used immediately after mixing to ensure optimum results.

REMEMBER

Acid perms are best suited to damaged, chemically treated, bleached or fragile hair.

TO DO

Briefly describe your salon's requirements for reporting stock shortages.

Preparation of client

TO DO

List the procedure for gowning and protecting clients for perming services in your salon.

It is best to gown up the client using a dark-coloured gown and disposable plastic cape as well as towels. In some cases, for example when carrying out a spiral wind, it is also advisable to use a drip tray to protect the client's clothes from chemicals. Barrier cream can also be applied to the client's skin around the hairline to help prevent any skin irritation.

Preparation of self

When applying perm lotion always wear gloves to protect your hands from chemical damage and skin irritation.

Preparation of tools and equipment

Before you begin your wind, have all the tools, equipment and products necessary for you to complete the perm on your trolley or work station; this will ensure that everything is readily available and within easy reach, and will help you to work more efficiently. Clean up work areas and dispose of any waste as you go along to help prevent accidents, minimise the risk of cross-infection and help to promote a professional image of yourself and the salon to clients.

TO DO

- List the three ways of sterilising equipment used in the salon.
- Check the manufacturer's instructions and your salon policy for information on the safe disposal of chemical waste.

TO DO

When seeking help from a colleague, clear instructions should be given. Read chapter 10, page 220 on training and development.

REMEMBER

Whether using conventional or alternative rods, **smaller rods give tighter curls**.

REMEMBER

Take into account any partings required when winding the top section.

Winding techniques

The following are examples of current and emerging perm winds.

Spiral winding

This method of winding has become very popular over the past few years. Spirally winding the hair gives a uniform, even curl along the length of the hair and is suitable for long, one-length hair.

Tools
Conventional perm rods, Molton Browners (available in foam and rubber), tubes and chopsticks.

Method
Divide the hair from forehead to nape into two sections of equal size.

The depth and width of each section to be wound depends on the amount of curl required.

For best results and maximum curl, take sections 1.25–2.5 cm (0.5–1 in.) deep.

The width of each sub-section will depend on the diameter of the rod used.

Method using Molton Browners (or equivalent)
Take a sub-section of hair and place end paper to cover ends of hair. Start winding from the bottom of the rod. Turn the rod, spiralling the hair up along its length. Once you reach the hair roots, bend the rod over to keep it in place.

Once this first row is completed, continue to take further sections, working up the head in the same way.

Tip: Wind hair around end paper several times to prevent hair unwinding.

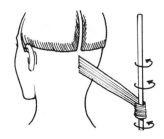 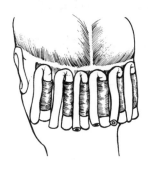

Spiral winding *Spiral wind in position*

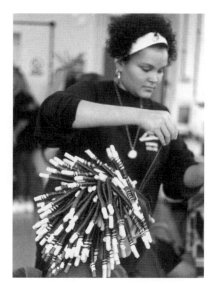 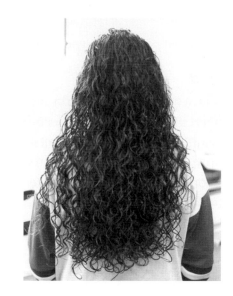

The rods in place *The result*

Stack wind

This perm wind is good for bob shapes in the hair to keep it flat on the top but with fullness at the bottom. The curls are mainly on the ends of the hair only.

Tools
Conventional perm rods and plastic sticks to keep the perm rods stacked.

Method
Start from the nape of the neck winding to the root.

As you progress up the head each roller is stacked on top of the other, winding further away from the root until the top section is only wound on the ends.

Hopscotch wind

This method of winding gives the hair texture, volume and varying curls, producing a non-uniform curl result, and is suitable for one-length hair or hair with long layers (see colour plate 5).

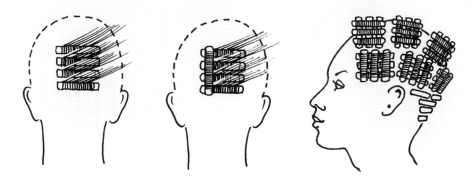

The hopscotch wind

Tools
Conventional perm rods, style formers (Wella), techniwavers (L'Oréal), rovalers (Wella).

Method
- Take a normal-sized section and weave thickly.
- Wind the back half of this section onto a rod.
- Continue in this manner until four or five rods have been wound, leaving unwound hair between each rod.
- Taking vertical sections of woven hair, wind so that the rod sits vertically on the previously wound section.
- Continue to wind all areas in the same way.

This wind can also be achieved simply by splitting a normal-sized section of hair and winding instead of weaving each section.

Piggyback wind

This method will give the hair texture, volume and varying curls, producing a non-uniform curl result. It is suitable for one-length hair or hair with long layers.

Tools
Conventional perm rods, style formers (Wella), techniwavers (L'Oréal), rovalers (Wella).

Note: To create varying curl strengths, different sizes, or types, of rods can be used.

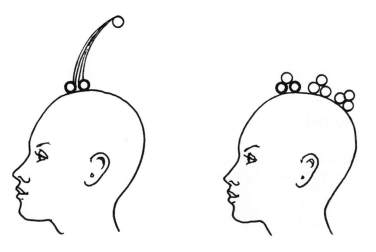

The piggyback wind

Method

- Take a fine section of hair and wind as for a basic wind.
- Take next section, but do not wind. Comb out of the way and leave.
- Take third section and wind as for first.
- Next, wind the middle section. This will sit on top of the previously wound rods.
- Continue to wind the remaining hair in the same manner.

This technique can be used on the whole head or in specific areas where extra volume is needed.

Note: Each section **must be fine**. If the sections taken are too thick, the centre rod will fall between the others and not sit on top.

Double/twin wind

This technique gives varying curls along the hairs' length, creating looser movement at the roots and curl along lengths and ends of hair.

Tools

Conventional perm rods work best.

Method

- Take section of hair and wind around rod.
- When half of the hair's length is wound, add another rod to the section and continue to wind both rods together down to the roots and secure.
- Continue to wind the rest of the head in the same manner.

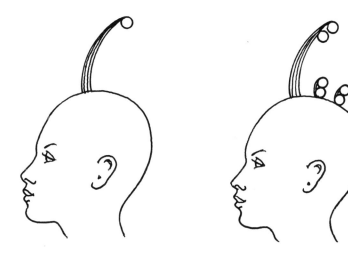

The double/twin wind

TO DO

Ask your product manufacturers/suppliers for information on new innovations for root perming, etc.

The following techniques are best suited for use on **short hair**, creating volume rather than curl. Various manufacturers have developed products especially for the needs of this type of client – for example Headlines by Wella, which gives style support and enables the service to be carried out more frequently than a conventional perm.

Weave wind

Gives root movement, volume and texture to short hair (colour plate 5).

Rods
Conventional, style formers (Wella), techniwavers (L'Oréal).

Method
- Take a normal-sized section of hair and weave thickly.
- Wind the back half of this section onto a rod, leaving the front part straight.
- Continue until all areas to be permed have been wound.
- Barrier cream can be applied to the woven sections which are not being permed to protect the hair from perm lotion.

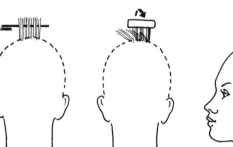

The weave wind

Pin curl perm

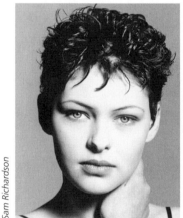

Pin curl perm

Gives the hair root movement, volume and texture (colour plate 5).

Tools
Lady Jane clips, either metal or plastic.

Method
As when setting hair using pin curls, sections can be square, oblong or triangular. Stand-up barrel curls will give root lift and volume, whereas flat barrel curls with a closed centre will give stronger curl movement.

Before starting, it is important to plan your wind, including the direction of curls and where volume is required, to ensure the desired result is achieved.

- Put end papers around hair points, form the hair into a pin curl and secure with a Lady Jane clip.
- Cotton wool can be put into stand-up curls to prevent them collapsing when lotion is applied.
- Continue to form curls on all areas of the head to be wound.
- A hairnet can be placed over the head during neutralising to protect the curls.

Barrelspring curl

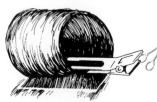

Stand-up barrel curl

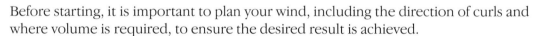

TO DO

Cut pictures from style magazines and describe how you could recreate each look. Include a description of the tools and equipment, winding techniques and products you would use on different types and lengths of hair.

Sam Richardson

Safety points to remember

- Make sure that the client is comfortable throughout the service.
- Check that perm rods are not causing discomfort and that there is not excessive tension on rods (loosen off perm bands).
- Applying lotion can be very dangerous, as it can easily run into the client's eyes. If this does happen, rinse immediately with cold water on a pad of cotton wool until the stinging stops.
- Always use a strip of dampened cotton wool around the hairline and hold a piece of cotton wool during lotioning to use for absorbing any excess.
- Pull burns may result if the hair is wound tightly – the neck of the hair follicle opens, allowing perm lotion to enter. If the scalp is scratched, this irritation could become infected, causing folliculitis.
- Do not use extra heat on sensitised hair as this will cause breakage.
- Many manufacturers' bottles of perm lotion and neutraliser look very similar. To avoid applying the wrong lotion, do not take out the bottle of neutraliser until you are ready to neutralise.
- When rinsing the hair make sure that the water temperature and flow are suitable for the client at all times.
- Familiarise yourself with manufacturers' instructions and your salon policy for the storage, use and disposal of perming and neutralising products. This is also covered under COSHH regulations 1992.

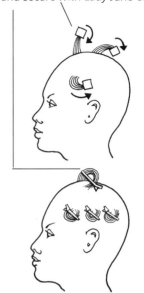

Form section of hair into curl and secure with Lady Jane clip

REMEMBER

- Make sure metal clips are coated or they will react with the perm lotion used.
- Perm lotions are available in cream or gel form which are more suitable for root perming.

Perming faults and corrections

FAULT	CAUSES	CORRECTION
The perm is not curly enough (weak curl).	Poor shampooing (hair greasy). Poor neutralising. Perm rods too large. Too few perm rods used. Perm lotion too weak. Not enough perm lotion applied. Perm lotion not left on long enough. Incorrect angling and placing of perm rods.	Re-perm the hair using a weaker perm lotion, but clip the rest of the hair well away from the perm lotion.
Hair too curly.	Perm rods used were too small.	May be gently relaxed if condition allows.
Overprocessed hair (looks frizzy when wet and straight when dry).	Perm lotion too strong. Too much heat used during processing. Too much tension used. Rods too small.	Suggest a course of conditioning treatments and regular haircuts. Do not re-perm the hair: it will break off.
Scalp/skin damage or irritation.	Perm lotion or relaxers coming into contact with scalp/skin – if it enters the hair follicle, 'pull burns' occur. Barrier cream not applied to sensitive skin areas. Cuts and abrasions to the scalp.	Remove any excess perm lotion with water. Apply a soothing moisturising cream to the area.

Cont.

FAULT	CAUSES	CORRECTION
Hair breakage.	Too much tension during winding. Rubber too tight or twisted. Perm lotion too strong. Hair overprocessed.	Suggest a course of reconditioning treatments or restructurants.
Band marks.	Rubbers placed wrongly on the hair. Too much tension.	Restructurant, deep-acting conditioner.
Deterioration of hair condition.	Overprocessing due to too many disulphide bonds being broken.	Restructurant, deep-acting conditioner.
Uneven result.	Incorrect sections. Uneven application of lotion and neutraliser. Uneven tension used.	Re-perm straight areas.
'Fish hooks' or broken ends.	Poor winding, ends not smoothly rolled around the perm rod.	These must be cut off.
Hair discoloured.	The neutraliser may have lightened the hair colour.	Apply a temporary or semi-permanent hair colour.

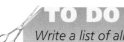

TO DO

Write a list of all the information that should be contained on a client record card.

Client record cards

When you have completed your perm always complete a client record card, giving full details of any products, tools, equipment and winding techniques used. If your salon uses a computer to store client details, re-read the section in Chapter 1 that deals with the Data Protection Act 1998.

TEST YOUR KNOWLEDGE

1   Why is it important to carry out hair and skin tests before and during perming processes?

2   What personal skills should you use when giving advice to clients?

3   Why should you consider the image of the client when perming?

4   What personal protective equipment should be used during perming? Why?

5   Why is it important to record and report stock shortages?

6   List three methods of sterilising tools and equipment.

7   Why is it important to work safely and keep work areas clean and tidy?

8   Under COSHH regulations, how should you dispose of chemical waste?

9   List the common perming faults and how to correct them.

10 List and describe a range of perming products available for use.

11 List the health and safety points to consider when perming hair.

Long layered styles

PLATE 1

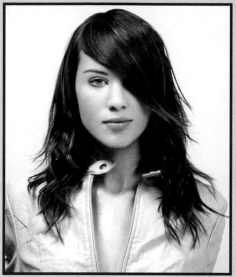

Style 1

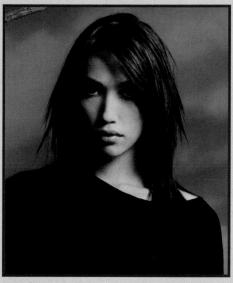

Style 2

Graduation variation step-by-step cut

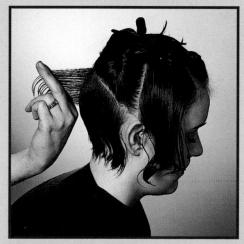

Step 1
Section above occipital bone. Starting at centre back, work parallel to head, cutting vertically into nape.

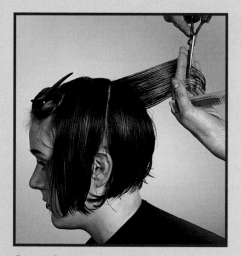

Step 2
Section from crown to top of ears. Continue working vertically, following guide from previous sections, working hair parallel to head.

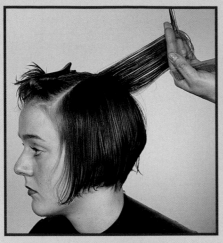

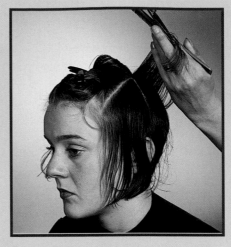

Step 3
Continue working through crown, lifting at 45° to create a gradual build-up of weight.

Step 4
Start working at same angle through side sections to front of ear.

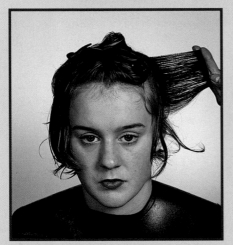

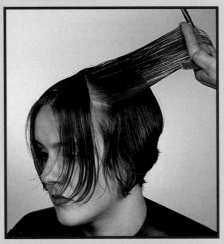

Step 5
Work with diagonal sections through sides and over direct back to maintain length and weight in front area. Repeat other side.

Step 6
Continue diagonal sections through to front area; blend remaining hair.

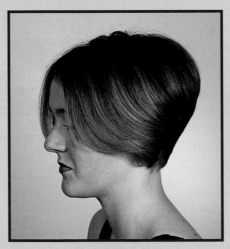

Step 7
Blow-dry with vent brush for smoothness and large round brush for fullness at crown.

PLATE 2

Textured layering step-by-step

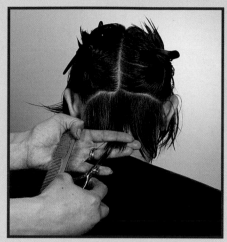

Step 1
Keeping length, texturise by cutting into each section about 2–3" deep. Keep control of hair to maintain balance.

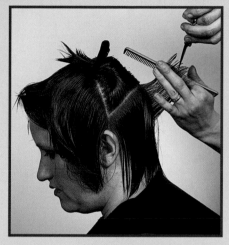

Step 2
Work technique through layering in the occipital bone area.

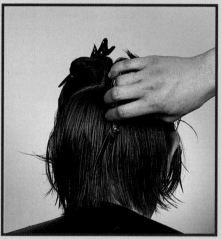

Step 3
When layering is complete, slice through hair to reduce weight.

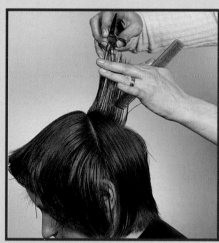

Step 4
Continue through crown, slicing hair to create a feathery effect.

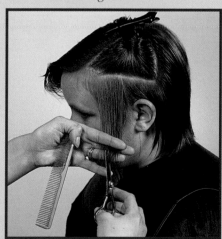

Step 5
Take a side section and using the same technique reduce weight and length.

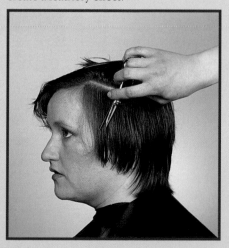

Step 6
Work as step 3. Repeat on other side.

PLATE 3

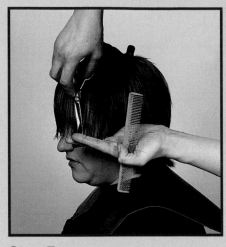

Step 7
Connect fringe with sides using same technique.

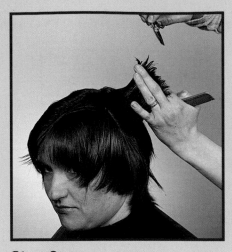

Step 8
Using guide from back, work textured layers through sides.

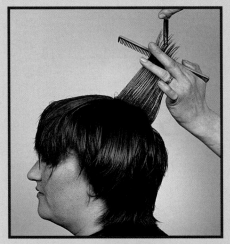

Step 9
Work same technique through crown.

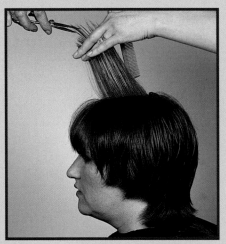

Step 10
Work layers through fringe area.

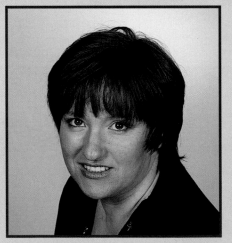

Step 11
Finger-dry back, smooth fringe with vent brush and use wax for definition.

PLATE 4

Perm winds

PLATE 5

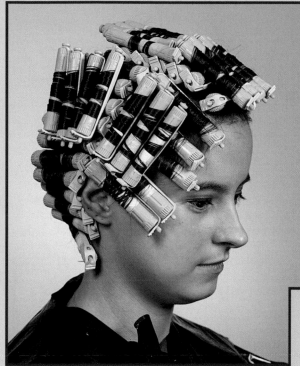

Hopscotch wind

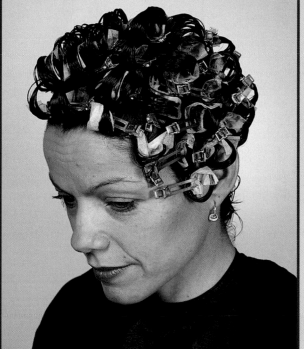

Pin curl wind

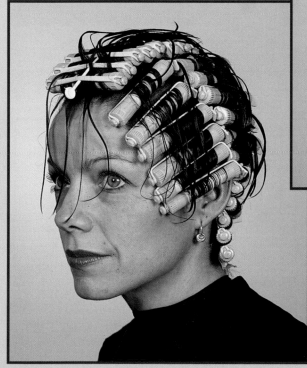

Weave wind

Random highlights step-by-step

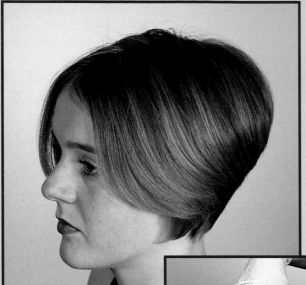

This technique is ideal for use on sleek, one-length hairstyles. The effect produced can be altered by taking larger sections to give a bolder result and using a variety of colour combinations.

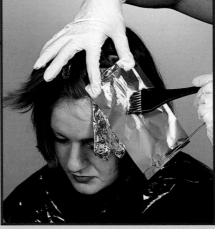

Step 1
Take zigzag section along scalp. Lift peak of inverted 'v' with pin-tail comb and separate from other hair. Place square of foil under hair strand and apply chosen colour.

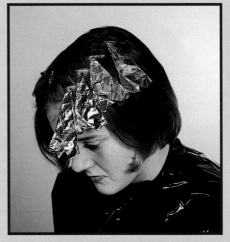

Step 2
Fold foil into a triangle-shaped packet to secure and prevent slipping. Repeat along zigzag section, colouring the peaks only.

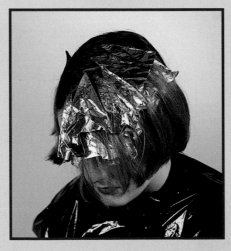

Step 3
Repeat the zigzag parting on next sections to be coloured and proceed as for steps 1 and 2.

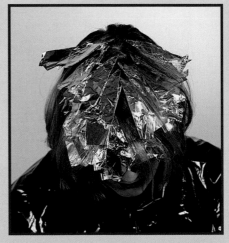

Step 4
Once completed, develop colour until desired shade is achieved, remove by shampooing and style.

PLATE 6

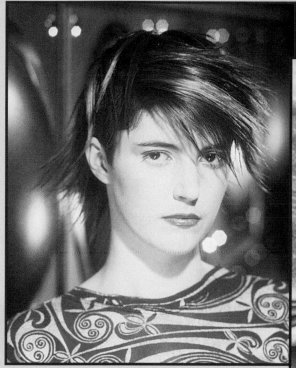

Block colouring

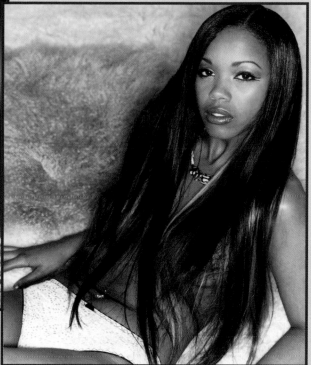

Hair extensions

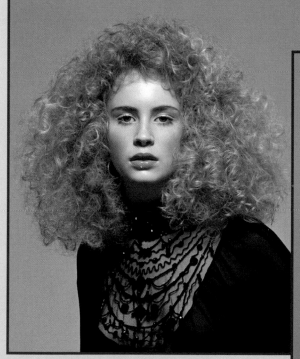

Alternative styling: Style 1

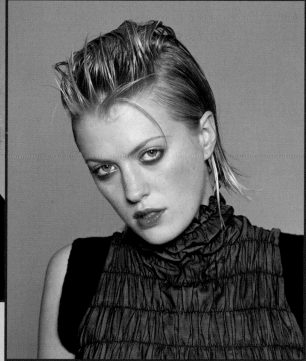

Alternative styling: Style 2

PLATE 7

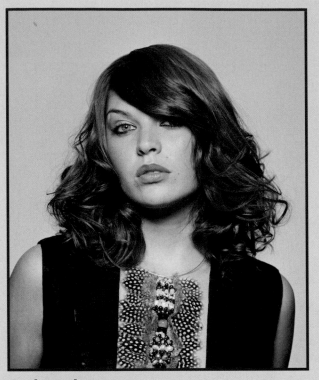

Curly style

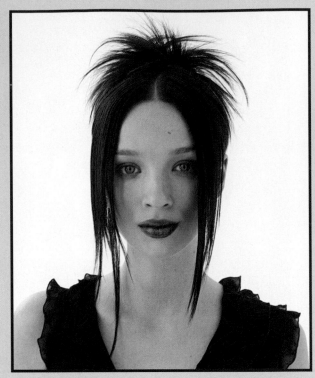

Classic styling

Twists and knots

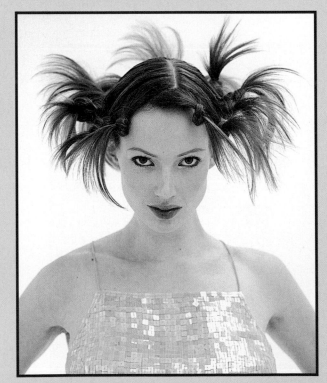

Style 1

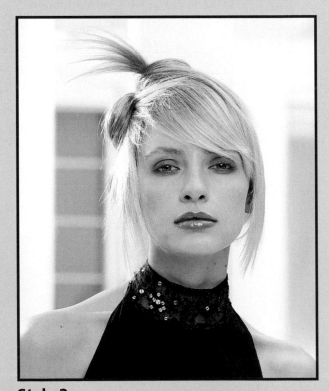

Style 2

PLATE 8

Chapter 7 African Caribbean hair

African Caribbean hair is unique as it can be moulded and adapted into many shapes. Like Caucasian hair, the type of look created can reflect the individual's taste in fashion, music and even religion. African Caribbean hair can withstand chemical processing over long periods of time without specialist care. This chapter is about salon services used especially for African Caribbean hair and will show you a variety of skills in relaxing, styling and dressing this hair type. Once perfected, these skills can be adapted and used on all types of hair.

This chapter covers the following NVQ level 3 units:
H31 Style hair using thermal techniques
H33 Provide corrective relaxing services
H35 Create complex styles using African Caribbean styling techniques
H36 Style hair using locksing techniques.

Characteristics of African Caribbean hair

Natural tight-curly African Caribbean hair can be quite difficult to manage as it has a tendency to tangle and become very dry. However, once it is straightened by either temporary or permanent means, it becomes extremely manageable and easy to style.

If you can offer services to African Caribbean clients such as relaxing, curly perms using heated equipment, conditioning (often called 'steaming' as the steamer is used to help conditioners to penetrate the hair), cutting, hair extensions and 'weave-ons', then your salon's professional image will be enhanced. You will also gain all the benefits of a greatly increased clientele.

African Caribbean hair structure

This hair is naturally dark because it contains more **melanin**.

It also needs more care and conditioning than Caucasian (European) hair because of its curly and crinkly shape. It tends to tangle easily, and may be damaged and break at the ends simply by being disentangled with combs and brushes.

Its curl is formed because of uneven keratinisation. This means that the keratin in the hair is more dense on the inside of the curl or wave – the 'para' cortex – and less dense on the outside of the curl or wave – the 'ortho' cortex.

African Caribbean hair may be:

- **Tight-curly**. If you look at the roots of the hair, you will see that it springs back curly near the scalp. Generally, tight-curly hair takes relaxer more easily.

- **Wavy**. If the hair is wavy at the roots, then it is generally stronger and needs a stronger relaxer.

- **Straight**. Ask the client if she has had a **relaxer** (a permanent straightener) or whether her hair has been **pressed** (a temporary relaxer).

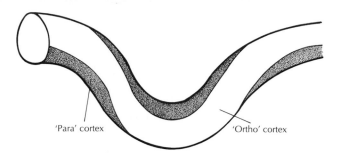

'Para' cortex   'Ortho' cortex

African Caribbean hair structure

TO DO

Re-read Chapter 1 regarding:
- *the texture of hair*
- *establishing hair condition (porosity, elasticity)*
- *hair structure, particularly the hair's cuticle, cortex and temporary and permanent bonds.*

African Caribbean hair has slightly more cuticle layers than Caucasian hair and is therefore initially more resistant to chemical processes such as tinting, bleaching, perming and relaxing. Because it has more cuticle it has less volume of cortex. This means that once chemicals have entered through the cuticle and into the cortex they will process African Caribbean hair more quickly than Caucasian hair.

HEALTH MATTERS

Make sure your client is correctly protected during thermal styling and relaxing by using the correct products, tools and equipment in accordance with the manufacturer's instructions, salon requirements and local by-laws. During consultations when you are examining the hair and scalp check for infections and infestations to reduce the risk of infecting either yourself or others in the salon.

Keeping your work area clean and tidy minimises the risk of cross-infection, maintains a professional salon image and allows you to work efficiently without disrupting other staff who may be working nearby.

Before you use it remember to check all of your electrical equipment for possible damage, loose connections and an up-to-date electrical safety test label to minimise the risk of accidents.

Styling African Caribbean hair with heated equipment

Shampooed and conditioned African Caribbean hair may be blow-dried and temporarily straightened by using a wide-toothed comb hand-drier attachment.

Wet hair can also be wrap set with a suitable blow-dry lotion/wrapping lotion or mousse to achieve straightness. Three rollers are placed in a downwards direction at the crown area, the hair is parted at the front (off-centre), brushed flat around the head and then dried under a hood drier.

Once the virgin hair is straight it can be moulded into shape by using either a pressing comb or heated tongs. Chemically treated (coloured, bleached or relaxed) hair that has already been processed needs greater care during thermal styling.

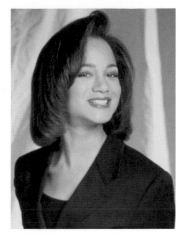

Temporarily straightened hair

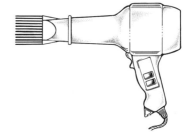

Drier with Afro comb attachment

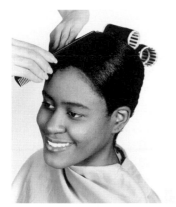
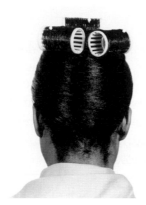
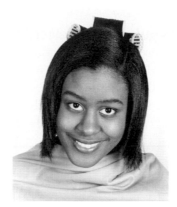

Pressing combs

Hair pressing or thermal hair straightening is a temporary process. It breaks the hydrogen bonds by using heat and tension.

The hair's natural water content or moisture is lost during this process, which is why pressing oils and thermal styling sprays are used to help replace this moisture. These oil-based products form a protective layer over the hair. They may contain silicones or long-chain hydrocarbons.

They are sprayed evenly onto each section of dry hair before pressing begins. Protective, moisturising scalp creams may also be used to prevent scalp dryness and these are applied with the fingers section by section before hair pressing.

Tight-curly hair in its unstretched state is described as being in an **alpha keratin** state. When the hair has been stretched straight by using heated styling equipment, it is in a **beta keratin** state.

Once the hair is dampened again, either by shampooing or as a result of the client perspiring or being caught in the rain, then the hair will revert to its natural curly **alpha keratin** state.

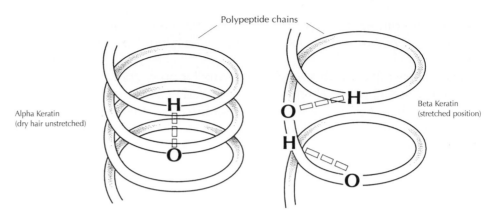

Alpha and beta keratin

Regular or non-electric combs

These combs are made of steel or brass with a wooden handle. They are heated by small electric heaters or gas stoves. Eight sizes are available, the space between the teeth varying – small teeth are used for fine hair, large teeth for coarse hair. Remember, the smaller the teeth, the more tension, which will create a straighter effect.

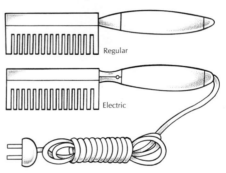

Pressing combs

Thermostatically controlled combs

These have a set working temperature.

Soft pressing

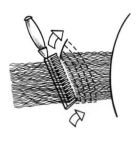

Before proceeding, always check the scalp for soreness caused by chemical treatments or scratches (from previous pressing or styling). Do not continue if this is present, but recommend conditioning treatments.

Using the following method, 70% of the curl can be removed.

Method

- Shampoo, condition and dry the hair.
- Apply a suitable pressing oil, thermal styling spray, pomade or cream to the hair and scalp to protect against scorching and add sheen.
- Take sections of 1.25 cm (0.5 in.), starting at the back and holding the hair at 90° to the head. Check the heat of the comb, then insert it 1.25 cm from the scalp.
- Slide the comb down the hair mesh, turning it over so that the back of the comb creates tension and straightens the hair.

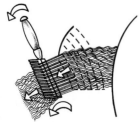

Inserting a pressing comb

- Comb each mesh of hair two or three times and gradually work towards the front.
- Once complete, apply a dressing cream, brush it through and style with curling tongs.

Hard pressing

This method removes almost all of the curl but is more damaging to the hair than soft pressing. Simply repeat the soft pressing method or straighten the hair again with Marcel thermal waving irons. These non-electric irons are slid down the hair mesh, pulling it straight.

Cleaning pressing combs

Always wipe the pressing comb free of grease and loose hairs after use. Clean combs work better, so use a commercially prepared product regularly to remove carbon build-up.

Thermal styling

Tongs can be used to produce a variety of effects, from curls and waves to ringlets or just for curling the ends of the hair (as in a bob). They are often used after blow drying the hair straight. Hot brushes and heated rollers can also be used to thermally style African Caribbean hair.

Many stylists who work with African Caribbean hair prefer to use tongs that are heated up in a separate heater. This enables several sizes to be available at the same time, to give a variety of styles and effects.

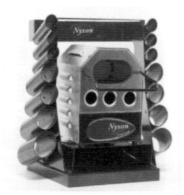

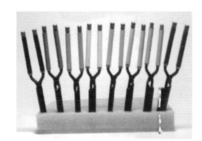

Afro tongs

Method for using tongs

The two movements used when tonging are:
- Opening and closing the tongs – which allows the tongs to move through the hair
- Turning the tongs – which curls the hair.

It is a combination of these two movements which can give the following effects:
- Waves
- Barrel curls or root curls

REMEMBER

- Check the heat of the pressing comb on white tissue or a white towel. If it scorches, let the comb cool down.
- Fine, bleached and tinted hair all need a lower comb temperature.
- Don't touch the scalp or skin with the hot comb or try to straighten very short hair – you could burn the client.
- Pressing normally lasts about 7–10 days but the hair will become curly again if the atmosphere is damp or the client's head perspires.
- No chemicals are used in these processes, so the hair can undergo pressing once a fortnight without undue damage. However, if you wish to apply chemicals (such as a relaxer), then all traces of pressing must be removed first (e.g. by shampooing).

REMEMBER

Always use a thermal styling spray before tonging to protect the hair from the heat of the tongs.

- Spiral curls
- Off base or end curls.

Always smooth the hair first by placing the tongs at the roots, gripping the hair, then sliding down the hair mesh a few times. This both smoothes the cuticle and allows you to establish a firm grip on the hair with the tongs.

Problems associated with thermal styling

Burns

- **Burns of the hair.** Remember always to use a lower temperature on fine, bleached, tinted and chemically treated hair.
- **Burns of the scalp or skin.** Always check the temperature of the irons on either a white tissue or a white towel. If it scorches or leaves a brown mark, allow the equipment to cool down before use.

Traction alopecia

Excessive tension used when hot-pressing hair by pulling at the hair shaft can lead to hair breakage or loosening of the hair in the follicle, causing traction alopecia. This baldness can become permanent if traction or pulling is carried out over a long period.

Cicatrical alopecia

This is a permanent bald patch where the hair follicles have been destroyed. It can be due to scarring from a heat burn, from thermal styling or even from a strong chemical relaxer left on the scalp for too long.

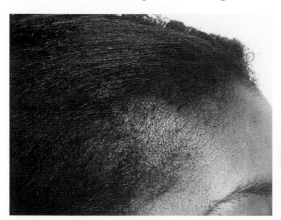
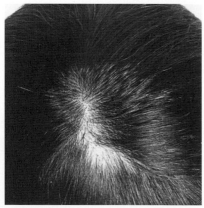

Traction alopecia   Cicatrical alopecia

THERMAL STYLING DIFFICULTIES AND CORRECTIONS	
Difficulty	**Correction**
Hair scorched	Recheck the tool temperature on white tissue before use
Very short hair	Use thermal oil spray on the scalp and avoid touching the scalp with heated equipment
Possible hair breakage	Cut the hair if possible, advise deep conditioning treatments to add moisture and protein before continuing

Electric tongs

Precautions when using tongs

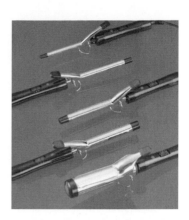

- Always pick them up by their handles.
- Always place a comb between hot tongs and the client's scalp when you are working near the scalp.
- Always use the stand or rest attached to the tongs to prevent work surfaces from becoming scorched, and plastic surfaces (such as equipment trolleys) from melting.
- Never put hot tongs into your tool bag. Allow them to cool first.
- Remember to switch the tongs off as soon as you have finished using them – it helps to prevent accidents.
- Light-coloured hair can be discoloured and scorched by the tongs, so do not have them too hot or use them for too long on the hair.
- Flexes can become twisted and insulation can gradually wear away, making the tool dangerous. Flexes must be checked regularly.

TEST YOUR KNOWLEDGE

1 Describe the following health and safety considerations:
   - Client preparation
   - Use of personal protective equipment
   - Cross-infections and infestations
   - Electrical equipment checks.

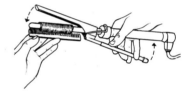

Using electric tongs

2 Why does African Caribbean hair need more care and conditioning than Caucasian hair?

3 Sketch and label a diagram to show the African Caribbean hair structure.

4 Which bonds in the cortex are broken by thermal styling?

5 Describe the equipment needed to thermally style hair.

6 What happens to the water in the hair during thermal styling?

7 How should you test the temperature of thermal styling equipment?

8 What could happen if you failed to test the temperature of thermal styling equipment?

9 Describe the products needed to keep the hair and scalp in good condition during thermal styling and how to use them.

10 Describe the reasons why soft pressing is more suitable for chemically treated hair and hard pressing is more suitable for virgin hair.

11 Describe how to prevent burns to:
   - the hair
   - the scalp or skin

   during thermal styling.

12 Describe traction alopecia and its causes.

13 Describe cicatrical alopecia and its causes.

14 Describe three potentially difficult problems which may occur during thermal styling and how you could correct them.

Relaxing

Relaxers are very popular with clients who have excessively curly or wavy hair because once their hair is permanently straightened they have a much wider choice of hairstyles. It allows the hair to be more adaptable and easier to manage. Relaxers may be applied:

- to virgin hair
- to the regrowth of previously relaxed hair
- to correct an uneven result from a previous relaxing treatment.

Tight-curly African Caribbean hair has more cuticle scales and is initially more difficult to chemically process evenly due to the speed of relaxing products.

Relaxing creams are extremely alkaline, with a pH of 10–14, which means they are very strong chemicals. Sodium hydroxide relaxers (caustic soda, sometimes called **lye**) are the strongest and fastest-acting chemicals.

Calcium hydroxide (occasionally potassium hydroxide or guanidine hydroxide) relaxers (sometimes called **no-lye**) are not as strong, but are gentler on the scalp and tend to lighten the colour, causing a reddish tinge. They are not as effective as other relaxers and do not require the scalp to be based. These relaxers are often available for home use, but they leave the hair dry and brittle.

Both of these straightening chemicals permanently change the structure of the hair by changing one-third of the **cystine** bonds into new **lanthionine** bonds (with one sulphur atom), which keep the hair straight. This process (sometimes known as **hydrolysis**) is stopped by a neutralising shampoo. The low pH of this shampoo stops any further chemical action.

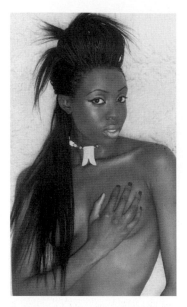

Relaxed hair

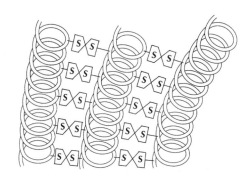

Tight-curly/wavy hair with disulphide bonds intact

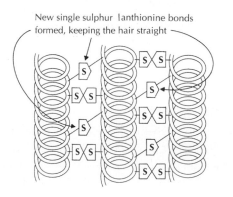

New single sulphur lanthionine bonds formed, keeping the hair straight

After being shaped with relaxing cream, processed and neutralising shampoo applied

The Cosmetic Products (Safety) Regulations 1989

These cover the rules that recommend different volumes and strengths of hydroxide-based products, i.e. hydrogen peroxide (which is mixed with tints and bleaches and is an ingredient in some perm neutralisers) and sodium, calcium and potassium hydroxide (relaxers). Product strengths will vary between those made for professional and non-professional (i.e. retail) use.

You can check the product strengths from the manufacturer's instructions and guidance notes. Further guidance can also be obtained by contacting the individual manufacturer or by contacting the Hairdressing & Beauty Suppliers Association (HBSA) at 1st Floor, Manfield House, 1 Southampton Street, Covent Garden, London WC2R 0LR, tel. 020 7836 4008.

Neutralising shampoos for relaxers

- Rinse the hair thoroughly to remove excess relaxer from the hair and scalp. Now apply the shampoo to the hair, remembering to use gentle massage techniques. Ideally the palms of the hands should be used so as not to irritate the scalp. This is especially true if the scalp has been irritated in the relaxing process.
- On the second shampoo, leave for five minutes, then rinse thoroughly.
- Check the manufacturer's instructions: some products change colour to show that the neutralising is complete.
- Blot the hair, then use a pH-balanced moisturising conditioner (to restore the hair to its normal acidic level) then rinse thoroughly.

The key factors of neutralising shampoo are that they:

- cleanse the hair of remaining relaxer
- restore the PH balance of hair
- close the cuticle.

Examining the hair and scalp

1. Check the client's scalp for any soreness, cuts, abrasions or disorders. If in doubt, do not proceed. If the client has an itchy or flaky scalp, then it is likely to be sensitive and may need a no-lye relaxer. Clients with a build-up of shampoo and conditioning products on their hair should have their hair shampooed five days before a relaxing treatment. Leave 1–2 weeks between tinting/bleaching and relaxing treatments.
2. Check the client's hair condition for:
    - Elasticity and tensile strength (elasticity test)
    - Tightness of curl (strand test, i.e. product strength and timing)
    - Texture and porosity (porosity test)
    - Previous chemical processes (incompatibility test)
    - Any breakage (elasticity test)
    If you are in any doubt, proceed with the necessary test and suggest some reconditioning treatments.
3. Check the client's record card for any previous treatments prior to service.
4. Check exactly what degree of straightness the client requires (use photographs from style books to give an indication of the finished result required).
5. Select a pre-relaxing treatment when relaxing porous hair. These products contain protein hydrolystates which cling to the hair and even out the porosity along the hairshaft. They are most effective on the cuticle layer.

REMEMBER

Neutralising shampoos work differently from perm neutralisers.
Never use a neutralising shampoo after a normal perm, or a perm neutraliser after straightening hair.

TO DO

Re-read the sections in Chapter 1 on strand tests, elasticity tests, porosity tests and incompatibility tests (pages 23–25).

REMEMBER

Relax only the regrowth area of bleached, highlighted or permanently coloured hair to avoid hair breakage from over-processing.

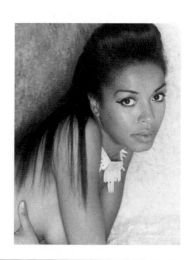

Matching relaxer to hair type

Relaxers are very strong chemicals.

- Make sure that you have sufficient product knowledge before using them. Try writing out the manufacturers' instructions in your own words.
- Make sure that you are using the correct straightening chemical for the hair, and the correct strength of chemical.

Sodium hydroxide (lye) relaxers

Nowadays these are oil based and leave the hair with body and shine. Look at the amount of curl in the hair by parting it – the more resistant curl formation is an important factor when choosing strengths of a relaxer. For example, coarse, tight-curly, virgin hair may need a super relaxer – normal curly hair may need a regular relaxer.

Benefits of using sodium-based relaxers are:

- Maximum straightness
- No need to mix
- Choice of different strengths
- Shiny results.

A choice of strengths is available (with a pH range of 12–13):

- For fine, tinted or lightened hair (hair that has been previously chemically treated, fragile hair) use mild relaxers
- For normal, medium-textured curly hair use regular relaxers
- For coarse-textured, resistant wavy hair use strong or super-relaxers.

Calcium hydroxide (no-lye) relaxers

No-lye relaxers may not necessarily be calcium hydroxide: sometimes the active chemical ingredient is potassium, guanidine or lithium hydroxide.

Calcium hydroxide relaxers are more suitable for clients with a sensitive scalp because they are not as strong as sodium hydroxide (lye) relaxers. This is the reason why no-lye relaxers are more often available for retail use.

Calcium hydroxide (no-lye) relaxers are mixed with an activator, and once mixed must not be used after 12 hours.

Benefits for selecting calcium-based relaxers are:

- less irritation
- ideal for scalp sensitivity
- useful for clients who are sensitive to sodium hydroxide.

TO DO

Take cuttings of tight-curly and wavy hair and strand-test them with a sodium hydroxide and calcium hydroxide relaxer. Make a note of the development times and any differences in the elasticity and condition of the hair. This will help you to determine which relaxer is best suited to the hair.

To base or not to base?

Always read the manufacturer's instructions regarding basing the scalp. Most sodium hydroxide relaxers do need a protective basing cream.

If the client has a sensitive scalp you should choose a calcium hydroxide (no-lye) relaxer, which does not require a protective basing cream.

Protection of the client and hairdresser

- Always wear rubber gloves, and gown up your client properly.
- Protect the client's hairline and scalp by applying protective base (or Vaseline) or special basing cream.
- Do not shampoo the hair or brush the scalp. If the scalp is sensitive apply protective basing cream (or Vaseline) to the scalp area section by section (like a tint). Place the cream, do not press or rub it in, as it must not cover the hair.
- Check the manufacturer's instructions. If a pre-relaxer treatment (filler) needs to be used, apply it evenly at this stage and blot off any excess.
- If the relaxer accidentally enters the eye it could cause blindness, so shield the unaffected eye with one hand, and flush the affected eye with lots of water. Seek medical help if the irritation persists. If the product comes into contact with the client's skin or clothes, flush the area immediately to dilute and remove the chemical.
- Always try to work in a ventilated area so that the fumes are less hazardous to both you and the client; it is your responsibility.

Choice of tools

Relaxer may be applied using different applicators such as brushes, combs and the hands. There are several effects on the hair and scalp. After a consultation you would need to select the appropriate method to meet your client's needs.

REMEMBER

Never mix relaxers, neutralisers and other products from different manufacturers – to achieve best results products of the same system must be used as they work in conjunction with each other. These are also manufacturer recommendations.

REMEMBER

Relaxers are hazardous materials as defined by the COSHH Act 1988 (see Chapter 2). They must not come into contact with the client's eyes or skin.

REMEMBER

PPE regulations state the importance of protecting yourself and others from risking harm or damage to property.

REMEMBER

The client should remove glasses or contact lenses before relaxing.

RELAXER APPLICATOR	EFFECTS ON THE HAIR	EFFECTS ON THE SCALP
Brush	Methodical application Clean sections Less pressure on the hair	Bristles more likely to cause irritation
Back of the comb	Methodical application Kinder to the hair Clean sections More pressure on the hair Advanced technique	Kinder to the scalp
Hands	Quick Can be messy Less control Ideal for longer virgin application Uses less product	More difficult to get even coverage

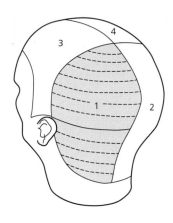

Regrowth application methods

With previously straightened hair, apply to the regrowth only, taking care not to overlap onto the previously straightened hair.

Section the hair into four and then prepare to apply the relaxer to the border of each section. Leave the front sections until last, especially the hairline as the hair and scalp tends to be more sensitive.

After you have applied the relaxer to the border of each section, start at section 1 at the back. Starting at the nape apply relaxer to small sections horizontally. Apply relaxer cream with the back of the comb or a brush, 6 mm from the scalp area to allow for product expansion. Work your way down to the crown. Complete sections 1 and 2 at the back, ensuring the hair is not touching the neck as the relaxer could irritate the skin. Then complete sections 3 and 4 at the front, working towards the front hairline. Apply to the front hairline, where the hair is more porous, last. The key to an even relaxation process is to ensure you apply adequate relaxer to the hair to ensure the hair absorbs enough of the product evenly. Ensuring the product is used economically will reduce the detrimental effects on the environment and increase salon profit.

Once the relaxer has been applied place the hair back into four sections. Cross-check the application in the opposite direction, reapplying relaxer to any uncovered areas. The product will swell during development. Once completed a strand test can be taken to determine the degree of relaxation. Use the back of the tail comb to remove some relaxer from a few strands of section 1. The relaxer should be removed from the root area only. Comb the hair straight gently, allow the hair to fall into its natural achieved straightness. Be careful not to irritate the scalp while carrying out this strand test. The strand test can be carried out on each section to ensure the required result has been achieved. Once the relaxation is achieved the relaxer can be removed.

Virgin applications

Remember that on virgin hair the relaxer needs to be applied to the lengths and ends first, then to the root area once the processing has started, so that the roots do not take too quickly because of body heat. When relaxing long hair, gloved hands can be used to spread the product through the lengths of the hair. The hands should be used to apply to the lengths only, as the heat from the hands can speed up the chemical process and if used on the scalp can also cause irritation.

Development and processing

Do not continually comb the hair – it will reduce its tensile strength and may easily break . Allow the hair to develop independently, continually checking the time to help ascertain how long the relaxer has been processing from start to finish.

Develop the product according to the manufacturer's instructions. This may take anything from two to 18 minutes. Check it continually by removing some of the product from a strand (strand test) and letting the hair relax with your comb to see the degree of straightness.

When processing is complete, rinse at a back wash basin with a strong stream of tepid water. Start in the same sequence as your application unless there is irritation in other sections then rinsing should start in this area first, after which you should return to the order of application. Let the force of the water remove the cream. Use your hands to lift the hair to help the removal process. Rinse until the water runs clear. Carry out

REMEMBER

Always check the instructions when using both relaxers and neutralising shampoos. They often differ from one manufacturer to another.

REMEMBER

High temperatures speed up the development process whereas low temperatures will slow it down.

a visual check of the hair and scalp as relaxer combined with pomades such as oil can be difficult to remove. It is important to ensure all products are removed from the hair to prevent over-processing. The timing in neutralising is also vital as it allows sufficient lanthionine bonds to be formed. Some manufacturers advise the use of a reconstructor at this stage, which should be left on for five minutes before the neutralising shampoo is applied. A post-relaxing treatment reduces the alkalinity in the hair, restoring the hair's normal pH and closing the cuticle scales. It is most effective in the cortex and is essential to restore the hair's pH to prevent breakage and close the cuticle.

Problems and corrections

Over-processing

If the product touches the scalp or skin for a prolonged period it will cause serious irritation, burning and damage. If the client complains of skin or scalp irritation during the relaxer process you should remove the relaxer from the area with an applicator and apply a protective barrier. If the relaxing process is completed and your client complains of irritation you should check that all the relaxer is completely removed with water, treat as a burn and seek medical advice. It is important to understand the different forms of discomfort your client may experience during the relaxing process. The following may be described by your client:

- increased body temperature
- itching sensation
- tingling sensation
- burning sensation.

If the product stays in contact with the hair for too long, the hair may become brittle, break off or even dissolve. Do not relax the hair if you think there will be any hair breakage.

Never use any additional heat (from hairdriers, accelerators or steamers) when processing sodium hydroxide relaxers – they develop very quickly and could dissolve the hair.

Corrections following processing

Over-processed hair will need a course of reconditioning treatments or restructurants. Do not attempt to re-process the hair – it is best kept regularly trimmed until the chemically treated hair has grown out.

The consequences of over-processing the hair can be detrimental to you as a hairdresser, and could result in:

- possible hair loss
- damage to hair
- inconvenience to the clients
- distress for the clients
- possible litigation
- loss of revenue.

Under-processing

If the relaxing product used was not strong enough, if it was incorrectly applied, resulting in roots, mid-lengths or ends being omitted, or if it was removed too soon, then the hair will still look crinkly and frizzy, resulting in different degrees of movement. There are many reasons for under-processing such as:

- insufficient processing time
- insufficient relaxer applied
- incorrect consultation
- incompatibility with previous products.

Leave sufficient time between relaxing and the corrective treatment (1–2 weeks). This is to ensure the hair is strong enough for the service and the scalp condition is suitable. A thorough consultation should be carried out to select the appropriate relaxer that may be applied to the **under-processed areas** of the hair (isolate the rest of the hair with a protective product).

The hair is then developed and the neutralising shampoo applied as normal to achieve perfectly relaxed hair that looks both straight and shiny.

Consequences of under-processing the hair are:

- hair is unevenly relaxed
- client is inconvenienced
- loss of revenue to salon
- salon image is damaged.

Corrections due to products

Corrective relaxing requires speed and caution alongside experience. A few key safety considerations should always be followed prior to carrying out this service:

- The timing of corrective relaxing will depend on the hair condition; ensure that manufacturers' instructions and your salon policy are always followed.
- Ensure you have personal protective equipment.
- Check client protection.
- Check the client's hair history.
- Check the client's hair condition.
- Client sensitivity to products.
- Questioning and recording your client's information to establish the previous products used on the hair is vital. Recording the response will help to provide reference for future treatments and also provide documentary evidence of the client's replies in case of litigation. It is important to check if your client has had an allergic reaction to treatments, is currently on or has recently taken medication. Any medical advice that would contraindicate a relaxing service must be discussed at the consultation stage prior to a relaxing service.
- Check you are aware of the correct handling and use of the products.

If a sodium hydroxide (lye) relaxer was used, then a weaker-strength product may be reapplied to the under-processed areas. Take great care with the application and constantly check the development.

If a calcium hydroxide (no-lye) relaxer has been used, which is a weaker chemical than the sodium hydroxide (lye), it may be that you did not check that the client's shampoos and conditioning products were removed from the hair beforehand.

Remember that calcium hydroxide (no-lye) relaxers tend to make the hair feel hard and clients are more likely to overuse conditioning products as a result.

It is possible to re-relax a no-lye treatment in the same way as a lye relaxer, but remember that calcium hydroxide relaxers can make the hair red. Reapplication of the product may increase this redness.

Effects of contraindications

CONTRAINDICATION	ACTION TAKEN
Skin sensitivities	Choose appropriate strength of relaxer
History of previous allergic reaction to relaxing products	Do not carry out the service
Skin disorders	May not be able to carry out the relaxer service
Incompatible products	Do not carry out the service
Medical advice or instructions	May not be able to carry out the service
Known allergies	Choose products appropriate for client

Record cards

Always keep your records up to date.

Relaxer Record Card

Client name _____

Address _____

Daytime telephone number _____

Pre-test results _____

Date of 1st relaxer _____	Date _____	Special notes _____
Colour treated/natural _____	Make of relaxer _____	_____
If treated, product used _____	Product strength _____	Neutralising time and method _____
Texture _____	Virgin head or regrowth _____	Conditioner _____
Condition _____	Result required _____	Result obtained _____
_____	Development time and method _____	Stylist _____

Other African Caribbean hair styling products

African Caribbean hair has a natural tendency to be dry, and when it is either thermally styled or chemically processed it needs a full range of conditioning products.

Shampoos

Shampoos for African Caribbean hair contain both mild detergents and a higher concentration of moisturising and detangling agents, creams and oils.

REMEMBER

Always allow sufficient time between relaxing and corrective treatments to minimise any damage to the hair.

REMEMBER

Hair in poor-condition is better set than blow-dried after relaxing.

REMEMBER

Never apply a sodium hydroxide (lye) relaxer over a calcium hydroxide (no-lye) relaxer in an attempt to re-process the hair. The no-lye relaxer deposits calcium in the hair and would act as a barrier.

Deep-acting conditioners

These are often oil based, adding moisture to the hair, and contain protein and polymer formulations to strengthen the hair. They must be left on for a minimum of three minutes, but most benefit by the addition of heat (either from a steamer or by covering with a plastic cap and placing under a drier).

Reconstructors

These help to replace proteins, amino acids and oils. They are sometimes used after the relaxer is rinsed off and before the neutralising shampoo is applied.

Moisturisers

These are sprayed onto wet hair to add moisture and body to the hair and to keep it wet during cutting.

Oil sheen sprays

These are used in the same way as thermal styling sprays on dry hair to give extra shine and finish.

Spritz, holding sprays and gels

These are all used for a finishing final hold on the hair.

TEST YOUR KNOWLEDGE

1 Which bonds in the cortex are broken by chemical relaxing?

2 Name the new bonds that are formed during the relaxing process.

3 Why is a neutralising shampoo used after relaxing?

4 Why is it not possible to perm relaxed hair?

5 What should you look for when examining the scalp before relaxing?

6 Describe the differences between sodium hydroxide (lye) relaxers and calcium hydroxide (no-lye) relaxers. How would you choose to use each?

7 Describe the three main types of sodium hydroxide (lye) relaxers.

8 Which type of relaxer needs a basing cream?

9 How should you protect your client before relaxing?

10 How should you protect yourself before applying a relaxer?

11 How does the COSHH Act 1988 relate to using relaxing chemicals?

12 During the application of relaxers describe how to:

- Section the hair
- Apply the product to virgin hair
- Apply the product to a regrowth
- Cross-check the application
- Develop the product
- Take a strand test
- Remove the product from the hair
- Use a neutralising shampoo.

13 What could happen to the hair and scalp/skin if the relaxer is over-processed, and why?

14 How could you rectify over-processed hair?

15 What does the hair look like if it is under-processed?

16 If a sodium hydroxide (lye) relaxer was under-developed resulting in different degrees of movement, how could you correct it?

17 Why should you allow sufficient time to elapse between relaxing and a corrective type of treatment?

18 Why could a calcium hydroxide (no-lye) relaxer be under-developed?

19 Why must you take greater care when correcting an under-developed calcium hydroxide (no-lye) relaxer?

20 What effect do different temperatures have on the relaxing process?

21 Why can you not correct a calcium hydroxide (no-lye) relaxer with a sodium hydroxide (lye) relaxer?

22 Why is a pH-balanced moisturising conditioner used after relaxing?

African Caribbean styling techniques

African Caribbean hair has the ability to be moulded and adapted for a variety of very different looks that are reflected in fashion and various trends. Demonstrating and perfecting twisting and plaiting skills will improve your already acquired dexterity, skills and knowledge.

Characteristics of African Caribbean hair related to complex styling

African Caribbean hair is naturally curly and requires more intense conditioning to keep it in good condition. It has to be treated with more care when brushing and combing as breakage can occur due to physical damage or neglect.

The cortex of African Caribbean hair is much flatter than that of Caucasian and Mongoloid hair and as a result it can absorb chemicals easily. This means that African Caribbean hair is more likely to suffer chemical damage.

HEALTH MATTERS

Hands

Plaiting and twisting over a long period of time may cause fatigue, arthritis in the joints and strain injury.

Ensure cuts on the hands are kept well covered until healed. Nails should be kept short so as not to irritate and hurt the client's scalp. Plaiting and twisting techniques, with extensions for additional hair, can be drying on the hands, so protect them with barrier creams and moisturisers. Hair products such as pomade, gels and oils (e.g. lanolin) can inflame contact dermatitis. This could permanently damage skin and nails and eventually affect your career in hairdressing.

REMEMBER

Ask open-ended questions to ensure you gain as much information as possible. Use pictures to confirm the finished look. Never be afraid to adapt your customer's finished look.

Consultation

Effective and clear consultation skills are the key to a satisfied customer.

Chemical products, plaiting and styling tools such as thermal tongs that are used on African Caribbean hair can be damaging to hair. It is therefore essential that you check the hair and scalp for hair disorders, breakage and physical damage.
The first signs of hair loss (traction alopecia) are:

- the hair becomes sparse
- hair becomes dull
- the hairline begins to recede
- the scalp becomes sensitive
- raised follicles.

TO DO

See Chapter 1 to find out about other forms of hair loss.

The area of traction alopecia must be treated with care – it is essential to avoid tension in these areas. Excessive tension used when twisting or plaiting can result in the client feeling uncomfortable. Damage to hair follicles and the first stages of traction alopecia can have long-term effects on the condition of the hair.

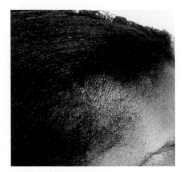

Traction alopecia

TYPES OF ALOPECIA	
Type	*Cause*
Traction alopecia	Excessive tension
Alopecia areata	Caused by trauma/stress
Alopecia universalis	A result of certain illnesses
Alopecia totalis	Caused by shock or stress
Cicatrical alopecia	Damage to the skin from severe cuts or burns
Post-partum alopecia	Reduced hormonal levels after pregnancy
Male pattern baldness	Hereditary
Diffuse hair loss	Hormonal

The type of alopecia will need to be considered when carrying out consultation prior to braiding/twisting.

Considering the client

With the desired look in mind, consideration of head and face shape and adapting the style to suit your client is vital for a good finished result. You must also have the ability to adapt your twisting technique to create a left- or right-side twist.

The client's hair density and texture must be considered. This is important when adding hair so that you can accurately work out how much hair to use and which texture is most suited to give a neat finish. As you work, keep checking how the added hair looks so that you can determine if it is well proportioned when plaited/twisted. If the hair is fine the style that is chosen may reflect this. Discussing your style and adapting your choice of style is essential in meeting the client's wishes.

The hair elasticity will determine the hair's strength. This will give you an indication of how much tension can be applied to the hair. Adapting the styles requested can minimise the damage. However, continued tension on the hair will lead to permanent hair loss.

Checklist

1   Check the client's scalp for hair loss (traction alopecia) in case you need to adapt your style.
2   Check the client's hair elasticity to determine how strong/weak the hair is prior to braiding so you don't apply too much tension on the hair.
3   Check the porosity and texture. You can then select the appropriate styling and finishing products.
4   Check for any previous chemical process that has been used, to ensure the hair will be blended smoothly in the finished look.

Client hair preparation

African Caribbean hair should be cleansed by using a pH shampoo with moisturising properties prior to plaiting or twisting. Using a penetrating conditioner will help to maintain the hair strength, preventing excess breakage during plaiting or twisting. Protect the client with a gown and towel. The scalp should be lightly based with a hairdressing pomade. Be careful not to apply too much as it may make it difficult to plait or twist.

Preparing yourself as a stylist

Try to estimate how long a service will take and be sure to allow for short breaks. Working with an assistant to complete the tail end of the plait or twist will help to reduce the time. Ensure you and your assistant plait and twist the hair with the same tension as differences in tension will affect the finished result.

Tools

Combs
You will need a comb to section the hair prior to twisting/braiding. This will ensure a neat finish.

Brushes
Prior to braiding and twisting the hair should be conditioned and brushed to spread products throughout the length of the hair.

Section clips
These will allow you to control the hair while twisting/braiding to ensure sections of the hair are not intertwined with other strands of hair.

When twisting or plaiting it is essential that sectioning is accurate, as this helps to control the hair. The style will also last longer, giving you the ability to achieve the desired look.

REMEMBER
Some plaiting or twisting techniques are not as durable on hair that has been treated with chemicals. The hair may not blend in the braid twist as neatly as it would if it had been chemically straightened.

Styling and finishing products

Gel/wax
These are usually packaged in tubes or containers and create shine. They can also be used to control the hair by keeping it firmly in place. Some gels give the appearance of a wet look. Others can be very drying on the scalp. Be sure to apply only to the hair.

Sprays
These are used primarily to give shine and control to the hair.

Oils
Oils used on the hair give it a shine and help to restore moisture. They also give the hair protection against harsh and long-term braiding.

All of the above products can be used before or during braiding/twisting. Care must be taken as they can make the hair very slippery, especially when attaching extensions.

Different styles

Full head
The entire head is plaited/twisted to give the finished effect.

Partial head
Completing the crown area only would be regarded as partial. Incorporating the twists/braids as part of the overall look is considered to be a partial head.

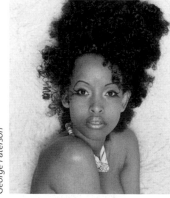

George Paterson

Classic
A classic look is a style that can be worn over a long period of time, regardless of age, fashion or trends of the time, such as a bob, pony-tail etc.

Sculptured styles
These are complex styles that incorporate design and different techniques to give the overall finish. They are often worn for special occasions or even hair exhibitions.

Additional hair
Styles can be created by using extensions to twist or plait. Extra care must be taken to prevent the hair falling on the floor and causing a slippery surface for colleagues and clients.

Using the products and hair extensions economically will increase the salon's profits and minimise waste. It is also important to avoid a build up of products in stock, as fashion trends change quickly.

Additional hair should not be cut with professional scissors, as the hair may not be real. It is still important to ensure the scissors are sterilised to stop the spread of infection and maintain a professional salon image.

Extensions can be twisted, burned or sealed with an elastic band, placed at the ends. Care must be taken when burning the ends of the extension – allow the hair to cool prior to twisting it. Elastic bands should be silicone based to protect the hair.

When dividing the hair prior to use, care should be taken to reduce wastage by holding the bundle of hair in the middle, with one hand. Using the other hand, divide from the centre and separate from the centre out firmly.

Twisting techniques

Two-stem twist

The two-stem twist is also known simply as **twisting**.

Achieve it by taking two equal-sized strands of hair and wrapping them across each other with even tension until all the hair is completely twisted together. The ends can be secured by using rubber bands or gels or waxes, which, used throughout the hair, will allow the hair to cling together and be held in place.

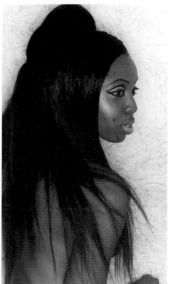

Comb twist off the scalp

The comb twist off the scalp is also known as a **gel twist**. These are individual twists that are created by using gel and the end of a tail comb. To create this look:

- Section the hair into approximately 1.25 cm (0.5 in.) squares.
- Apply a strong gel, which will not flake in the hair when dry. Comb the hair through thoroughly to distribute the gel from the roots to the end.
- Using the end of a tail comb, rotate the comb in the hair so the hair is wrapped around the comb.
- Continue this movement pulling the tail comb in a downwards direction as you pull the hair downwards. Take your sections in a brickwork method so no obvious lines appear when finished.
- To finish, the hair is allowed to dry by placing the client under a warm drier for 30–40 minutes depending on length.
- Apply a gloss spray to add shine to the hair.

Maintenance: use a scarf to cover hair at night and for control. Continual use of oil sheen sprays is necessary, but do not use heavy pomades as this will unravel the twist.

Senegalese twist

The Senegalese twist is very similar to a two-stem twist.

- To begin, select your section depending on how thick or thin you would like your twist to be.
- You may need to practise this method prior to attempting a finished look.
- Separate the hair into two individual strands containing even amounts of hair.
- Twist one section of hair between your fingers; now, holding the strand of hair twist the other section of hair both in a clockwise movement.
- Place one strand over the other strand with even tension to create a neat lock; continue until you reach the end of the twist.
- The ends of the twist can be secured by using an ornament, such as a pearl, or string.

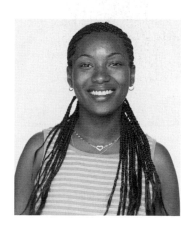

When selecting the setting for a Senegalese twist, your twists should be made in the direction you wish the hair to lie. The complete twist should give the impression of a 'rope' entwined together evenly.

This look can be worn casually or dressed up for an evening occasion.

Maintenance: gently apply a light pomade to maintain hair and scalp.

George Paterson

The use of an oil spray will add gloss to the hair.

Duration: this varies depending on whether extensions were used; if so, then it can last up to 2–3 months, if not 1–2 weeks.

Flat twist/ comb twist on the scalp

To create this look the hair needs to be smooth/straight, as a flat twist sits parallel to the head.

- The section of hair used is a narrow channel, sectioned neatly to achieve a neat finish.
- Evenly separate the hair into two strands. Wrap one strand over the other strand of hair keeping the hair flat to the scalp. A rotating movement must be used while wrapping each section.
- A twisting movement is used as you pick up the next piece of hair along the channel of hair.
- Again wrap the hair over each other once, keeping it flat to the scalp. Ensure you have even tension while twisting and folding your section.
- When you have completed your section on the scalp, the ends of the hair can be secured by using a silicone band. This is to ensure the flat twist cannot unravel.
- The hair can now be dressed by tonging or blow-drying into the remaining hair.

Maintenance: use an oil sheen spray to give gloss and shine. Cover at night using a light scarf.

Durability: usually one week.

Corkscrew twist

This twist is much thicker than the average twist. The corkscrew effect is defined by using a strong thread to separate each individual twist. The thread selected should be as close to the natural hair colour as possible.

- Take a 2.5 cm square (1 in.) section of hair.
- Take a piece of strong thread (approximately twice the length of the hair).
- Attach the thread to the base of the hair. The thread should hang like a loose tail.
- Separate the hair into two even strands.
- Wrap the thread around as you twist the two sections of hair together.
- Continue until you have completed the section.
- Hold the string and push up from the bottom until it puffs into a corkscrew effect.

Maintenance: place a scarf over the head to control the hair. Also, use a pomade to help keep the hair and scalp moist.

Duration: with extensions, this can last for up to 2–3 months.

Plaiting techniques

Tree plaiting

Tree plaiting is a variation of a three-strand plait allowing the hair to be left from the main stem of the plait. The sections that have been left out are then styled by tonging or using styling products such as gels or waxes, and can create an image of a tree (the hair is left out from the stem, being the branches of the trunk).

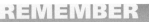

REMEMBER

Use a silicone band so as not to cause damage or breakage to the hair.

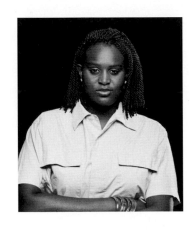

Tree plaiting off the scalp

- Take a section of hair as you would for a single three-strand plait. Separate the hair into three, even, separate strands of hair.
- Place the right side section under the centre section.
- Then place the left-hand side of the hair under the centre section.
- Place the strands firmly under the centre sections so a clear definition can be seen.
- Repeat the first two stages again.
- Prior to crossing the left side under the centre section again separate a few strands of hair and leave out of the main stem.
- Place the hair under the left-hand side under the centre.
- Repeat on the right-hand side.
- Alternate the sides where the hair has been left out. This will allow the finished look to be balanced.
- Repeat on the right-hand side, leaving a few strands of hair from the main channel on that side.
- Repeat on the left-hand side.
- When you have completed the plait it can be dressed as you wish.

Tree plaiting on the scalp

This technique follows the same principles as a tree plait off the scalp, but the initial plait starts parallel to the scalp. The technique is the same as for a corn row, but with strands of hair left out like the branches of a tree.

- To start, take a channel of hair. The size will depend on your finished look.
- Divide the hair into three even strands of hair. Place the right strand under the middle strand and place the left strand under the middle strand.
- Again place the right strand under the middle strand but now merge some hair from the side of the channel of hair with the right section you have taken.
- Proceed to do the same on the left-hand side. Combine hair from the left channel into the strand you are placing under your middle section.
- Repeat on the right-hand side.
- When you have completed an inch along the length of the channel, remove a few strands. This will create the effect of the branches of a tree.
- Alternate this technique so the finished braid is even and balanced.
- When the plait is completed it can be secured by using ornamentation or silicone bands.

The goddess braid

The goddess braid is usually much larger than most braids. Planning of the finished look is important to create the design. Using additional synthetic (rather than human) hair will provide the necessary weight and reduce the cost.

The goddess braid is usually done to create an elegant evening look.

- To start the braid, place the hair into two sections, one at the front and one at the nape.
- Select the amount of synthetic hair you wish to use. This will depend on the size of your section. Divide this in half to form a U-shape.

- Take a section of natural hair about 10–12 cm (4–5 ins) vertically.
- Place the hair extension over the natural hair holding it at the roots.
- Hold the hair at the point where the two pieces sit on top of each other in the centre. Separate the hair into three strands holding them firmly in place.
- Now place the right-hand strand over the centre strand and equally separate the hair. Each time you do this you pick up some hair from the same side of the section you are braiding.
- Repeat the same procedure on the left-hand side ensuring a small amount of natural hair is added each time you cross over.
- Ensure the natural hair is concealed with the synthetic hair while you are braiding.
- When you have completed the one side you can use the same technique to braid the other side of the head.
- The ends are braided in the same three-strand plait and the hair can be twisted and secured up above the head depending on the pre-planned design.

Aftercare

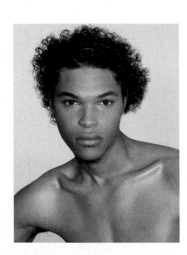

Looking after hair which is twisted or plaited can be done with a combination of methods, depending on the natural hair needs. Use of an oil-based product is very effective as African Caribbean hair thrives on oils.

- Rosemary oil – helps to remove tangles in the hair
- Olive oil – is good for conditioning
- Sage oil – smoothes an itchy scalp
- Jojoba oil – good as a skin moisturiser and also helps to remove hardened sebum.

These oils are good to use and can be mixed with base oils, as some can be quite potent. They are used as hot oil treatments to maintain the natural hair.

Shampooing hair which has been twisted/plaited with extensions can be carried out in the normal way. A little rotary massage technique should be used so as not to disturb the finished look. You may find that you will need to shampoo the hair three times to remove a build up of products and sebum. Choosing a professional product will reduce the drying effect that harsh shampoos have on African Caribbean hair.

Shampooing hair that has been twisted/plaited without extensions tends to loosen up braids when they are wet. It will tighten again when it dries, thus making the hair look untidy. It is much more difficult to remove braids that have been shampooed in this way. This is because the water tends to encourage the hair to matt. Therefore, these styles are designed to be worn for 5–10 days and then removed.

Once shampooed the hair can be towel-dried gently and placed under a warm drier or left to dry naturally.

Applying a light pomade to the scalp will ensure the scalp condition is maintained. The use of braid sprays on braids is a good way to moisturise the scalp. They can minimise itching and will also put a sheen on the hair, as they are silicone-based products. These products should be used in conjunction with other forms of aftercare methods, as they can be short lived.

ADVANCED HAIRDRESSING

At night the hair can be maintained by covering the head with a scarf – this is for control and to maintain the finished look as long as possible. A satin or tightly woven silk scarf is the best choice, as it will smooth down plaits. Cotton scarves tend to absorb the protective oil placed on the hair.

Once the hair has been removed from plaits or twists it should be cleansed and conditioned using a penetrating treatment or a restructurant conditioner. This is to build up the hair's natural strength and to replenish any lost moisture. The general appearance will also be improved. More than one treatment may be necessary if the hair has been braided over a long period of time. This should always be undertaken prior to any chemical services being carried out. Over a long period of time additional hair will reduce the hair's natural moisture level and elasticity, leading to possible hair damage. Carrying out elasticity and porosity tests will help you to determine the hair's strength and ability to withstand a chemical process.

TEST YOUR KNOWLEDGE

1   List the products advisable for maintaining hair that has been plaited or twisted.
2   What aftercare advice could you give your client?
3   State a hair disorder that can be attributed to harsh plaiting over a long period of time.
4   Why is good posture essential when plaiting/twisting hair?
5   Why is it essential to carry out a full consultation prior to starting work on your client's hair?
6   What advice would you give prior to a chemical process if a client has had plaits in her hair recently?
7   What does African Caribbean hair thrive on?

Locksing

The history of locks

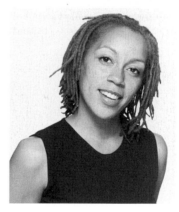

Many people assume that locks are worn for a spiritual or political reason. This may be true for some people, but many simply like them. The dreadlocks style of hair can also relate to a way of life that is known as Rastafarianism. Locksed hair is universal and it appears in many cultures in the world, for many reasons.

Africa is the birthplace of locksed hair – it can be traced back to an Egyptian goddess who wore her hair in spiralled coils. Today it is worn worldwide for individual reasons.

Considering locksing their hair represents a very important stage of the client's life. Most clients who locks their hair have tried chemical processes, relaxers, perms and various styles over the years and have reached a point where they want to be natural.

Hair grows for about three years before it goes into a resting phase and is shed from the follicle. Due to the fact that African Caribbean hair is curly, it appears to grow much slower. Also it can be shortened by breakage from sleeping in rollers, too much blow-drying, tonging etc.

Stages of locksing

Pre-locksing stage – 1 to 6 weeks
This is the initial stage of locksing. The hair is palm rolled into thin, tightly coiled spirals. The hair can be rebellious at times and care is needed to maintain it.

Growing stage – 6 to 8 months

The pre-locks will begin to explode in one spot like a bud. This process usually occurs about 2 cm (0.75 in.) down the locks from the roots. The locks begin to interlock and matt. The locks are directing downwards.

Final stage – 8 to 18 months

The locks are airtight interlocked and spiralling. The locks are solid, fairly tight and uniform in appearance.

Locksing your hair means no blow-drying, tonging, or physical damage. So many clients who locks their hair are happy with the length they can grow. When the curly African Caribbean hair grows undisturbed the strands intertwine with each other and form random matted hair. When hair is shed it is left in the hair, thus giving the appearance of matted hair. If the hair is left undisturbed it cannot be removed by combing. The only way it can be removed is by cutting.

Preparing the locks

The hair should be shampooed and conditioned prior to starting. The hair must be completely natural to start locksing. For maintenance some clients may wish to wear their hair in twists for some time while the hair is growing out of a chemical service, or until the hair is the length they require. This adjustment stage can be dealt with in many ways. Discuss with your client the various options available.

Tools and products needed

- A spray bottle containing water for damping the hair and to encourage it to coil
- A leave-in conditioner
- A comb to section the hair
- Sectioning clips to separate the hair with sections (the brickwork method is best to avoid the initial gap)
- Brushes – a brush may be needed to back-brush hair that is naturally straight to begin the locksing process. Brushes can be used to help spread the products throughout the hair length prior to beginning the locksing process.
- To begin, you may need a holding agent such as a gel or wax. These products help the hair to curl and hold together until the hair is locksed. The use of light products is advisable as they can be rinsed from the hair easily without disturbing the new locks.

Palm rolling

This method of creating locks is widely used in many salons today. Creating locks can take from six months to one year, and is done in stages: pre-locksing, the growing stage and the final stage. This method takes full advantage of the natural ability of the hair to coil together, and it is the gentlest method of locksing. It allows the cuticle scales to remain flat, and the hair is smoothed in one direction.

- To begin, the hair must be shampooed and conditioned. Keep the hair in its natural state and blot dry to remove any excess moisture.
- Take sections horizontally across the head in a straight line and separate the hair with a sectioning clip. Take a small square or triangle section of hair; the size depends on how small or large you want the locks to be. Apply a small amount of gel to the hair near the scalp area. Twist it once in a full clockwise rotation ensuring the twisting is close to the scalp. The gel will help the hair to hold together.

- Place the hair in the palm of your left hand and roll it by placing the right hand on the top.
- Tuck the ends of the hair near the thumb and fold the thumb down. This will keep the hair in place.
- Move your right hand towards the left-hand fingertips in a downward movement. Allow the hair to be removed near the thumb so it can also be rolled.

To complete a full head of short to medium-length hair could take up to one hour. Long hair could take 2–3 hours depending on the density. One individual palm roll takes five minutes.

Cultivated locks

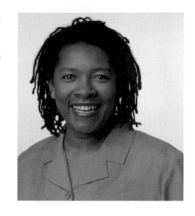

'Cultivated' describes locks that have been created naturally and left to develop without much intervention by the hairdresser. Naturally curly hair will have the ability to locks. Straight hair will do the same after some time, but it will not create true-coiled locks. The 'Rastafarian' locks, as it is known, will not matt together to form random individual locks through a natural process.

Once the hair has locksed together it can then be shampoocd. This should be carried out by using a little aggressive massage technique so as not to intertwine the locks created. The hair should be blot dried placing a towel over the head and squeezing out the excess moisture. Place the hair under a drier to remove all moisture. A light pomade may be applied to the scalp if needed to maintain the condition.

REMEMBER

Excessive oil can defeat the hard work of creating locks.

Hair which is naturally straight, wavy or silky may need to be back-brushed/combed prior to the locks being cultivated to allow the hair to matt together.

Wrapping technique

Silky locks

- To begin, the hair is shampooed and conditioned in the normal way. This form of locks is a braid with an extension that gives the impression of locks. The braids are individual plaits with additional hair added to the length and body of the hair.
- Synthetic hair is then wrapped from the base knot at the root area. Hold the hair and begin wrapping the extension around the braid in a spiral technique to the end of the braid. Synthetic hair will give a shiny finish (human hair can also be used).
- The ends are sealed by burning and rolling the ends between the finger. (This skill may require practice.)
- The finish will be silky and shiny without the matted finish.

REMEMBER

Allow hair to cool prior to rolling ends.

REMEMBER

When using added hair extensions, care must be taken to prevent wastage. This can be costly to the salon and cause hazards to others in the salon. Hair extensions can be very slippery on the floor.

Duration: silky locks could last up to three months.

Timing: short–medium-length hair density – one to three hours. Individual silky locks – five to 10 minutes each.

Yarn locks
This is similar to the silky locks method but the end result is a matt finish. It can give an alternative look to locks.
- To start, the hair should be shampooed and conditioned.
- Section the hair for a braid with extension.
- When completed each braid is individually wrapped with a single-ply of yarn from base to the end (special thread can also be used).

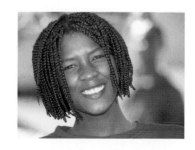

- The ends are burned and twisted by the finger (allow the hair to cool slightly prior to twisting).

Duration: this type of locksed braid will last for about three months.

Timing: this process takes the same length of time as silky locks.

When creating a silky or yarn lock, it is vital to select the closest match of added hair to the colour of the locks.

The correct amount of added hair is key to achieving a realistic finish of natural locks.

Full head/partial head

All these forms of locksing can be created on a full head of hair or used to create a style. Locksing only the crown area or the fringe is also possible. The remaining hair can be cut short to create the finished result.

Colouring natural locks is possible. All types of colouring products can be used. An increased amount of colour may be needed due to the bulk of hair.

Wearing accessories such as hair clips or beads can enhance the locks.

Hats or scarves can protect locks from the sun.

To locks or not to locks

There are some instances when locksing should not be carried out. Not all types of hair are suitable for this technique. For example, hair that is dry and brittle in texture would not be suitable for locksing. The lack of moisture resulting from by locksing would increase hair breakage. This is also true of fine or thin hair. The pressure on the hair would cause it to break.

If there are any cuts and abrasions on the scalp the palm-rolling technique would cause discomfort to the client, irritating the scalp.

Suspected infection/infestation – if a client is thought to have an infection of infestation no hair dressing should be carried out. The client should be referred to a general practitioner in all cases. Occasionally a trichologist may be recommended.

TO DO

Re-read Chapter 1 regarding hairdressing consultation and Chapter 2 regarding health and safety and security in the salon.

CONDITION	REFERRAL TO GP	REFERRAL TO TRICHOLOGIST
Eczema	✔	
Psoriasis	✔	
Alopecia acreata	✔	✔
Impetigo	✔	
Boils	✔	
Traction alopecia		✔
Folliculitus	✔	
Ringworm	✔	
Diffuse alopecia	✔	✔
Warts	✔	

Maintaining created and cultivated locks

Once the locks are formed the hair should not be shampooed for at least 3–4 weeks. This will help the hair to form the coil pattern. If shampooed before this time has elapsed, the hair may uncoil and you will have to re-twist the hair lock.

Instead of shampooing, use a moist cotton pad or swab with mild antiseptic skin cleanser. This is designed to lift grime and will also relieve any itching, providing you with the opportunity to delay the shampooing process. You may also use the swab on the exposed parting. Finish the cleansing with light oil and re-twist the new growth and locks that have become unfurled.

At night a scarf can be worn to keep the locks under control.

Shampooing the locks
Shampooing the locks can be carried out every two weeks. The use of a shower will make the process far easier.

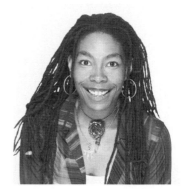

When shampooing concentrate on cleansing the scalp first. Smooth the shampoo down the length of the lock. Rinse the hair thoroughly. Rinsing the hair may take 3–4 minutes, as you must ensure all traces of shampoo are removed from the locks.

If the locks are shorter, rinse after a gentle shampoo. Covering the hair with a net before rinsing will help to protect the coiled hair at the ends. Once the hair is rinsed, squeeze any remaining moisture out with a towel. Do not rub the hair as this will disturb the coil formation and make the locks look untidy.

Conditioning
Locks are more manageable when they have been moisturised and conditioned. Adding oil to the hair will make it supple.

Use a leave-in conditioner with water-based consistency, as it will not be visible on the locks. Other moisturising conditioners may be used, but you must ensure they are removed from the hair. Hot oils are excellent conditioners for locks as they thrive on oil. Spray oils and hot oils are ideal for home use to maintain hair and scalp moisture.

Reconditioning the hair after locksing is vital to replace lost moisture and hair elasticity. It will also improve the hair's overall appearance. Locks can look very dull if not treated with care. Placing products on the roots first and spreading through the middle length and ends will ensure products are not wasted.

Removal of locks
Cutting is the only way to remove locks if the hair has been locksed for some time. The same conditioning technique may be used, but a series of reconstructants may be used to help strengthen and prepare hair for other chemical services. An elasticity and porosity test should be carried out prior to any chemical services to determine the strength and general condition, allowing you as the stylist to make the correct decision.

Re-twisting
Once the hair is conditioned, prior to drying, the new growth should be re-twisted at the roots through to the ends of the locks. To maintain the created effect, if a cultivated finish is required the hair is not twisted. The scalp can be lightly oiled with pomade to maintain it, prior to re-twisting. Using a gel or spray can help to re-twist the new growth, assisting it to intertwine with the existing locks.

Drying locks can be carried out by placing the client under a warm drier. Place a net loosely over the client's hair, and allow to dry. Do not over-dry the hair because the locks will feel brittle.

Using excessive repetitive tension on the hair, such as a tight pony-tail, can cause the locks to become thin. If continued this can lead to the first signs of traction alopecia. The first sign of this may be raised hair follicles and also client discomfort. The hairline may recede and look dull. Due to continued harsh treatment of the locks the scalp may become sensitive.

Repairing locks

Over a period of time locks can appear thin. This is caused by many things. As a hairdresser you must carry out a thorough consultation if this occurs and decide the best course of action for the individual client.

The following are some of the causes:

- traction alopecia
- male pattern baldness
- menopause
- extensions being too heavy for the hair
- the use of medication, e.g. for high blood pressure.

Hair extensions can be used to fill out thin locks or extend the actual length of the natural locks. In this case extensions are used as the starting point at the base of the locks. The extensions are used in the same way as for the yarn/silk lock. This will take the same time to master. Where the hair is thin, wrap the extension around the hair so it overlaps more to give the impression of being an even lock. End your locks with the extension wrapped past one end of the natural hair and burned and twisted to maintain the finished result.

Ensure the hair extension matches the natural colour of the locks as closely as possible. Also consider whether the required finish is matt or silky extension locks. Carefully check the texture of the extension and compare against the natural hair. When using extensions the tension used when attaching the hair will determine the balance and thickness of the extension on the natural hair. Even tension must be used throughout with an even balance of added hair. The size of the extension will depend on the locks you are attaching it to.

The extension can be removed and replaced after four weeks. If left longer the hair can become matted with the real locks and be very difficult to remove. Thinning of the locks can also occur when the new growth has not been re-twisted to maintain the finished result. So the weight of the locks will pull on the new growth if not intertwined together.

Wearing extensions in the hair for a long period of time will reduce the hair's moisture level. It is vital that oil-based conditioning treatments are used on the hair and scalp. This will improve the appearance, as over a period of time extensions will lose their natural look. Continual wearing of extensions will put extra stress on the hair's elasticity. Deterioration of the hair may result in referral of the client to a trichologist.

It may be necessary to cut the hair. Making regular visits to the salon for treatments such as oil treatments and leave-in conditioning may help improve the condition of the hair and the scalp.

TO DO

Practise this method of wrapping. Start with 1.25 cm (0.5 in.) of the thickness of the hair extension. Your braid should be half the size.

REMEMBER

When choosing extensions select an appropriate amount of hair to give the impression of the locks being even throughout their length.

TEST YOUR KNOWLEDGE

1. What are some of the first signs of traction alopecia?
2. List some hair conditions where locksing should not be carried out.
3. What are the three stages of locksing?
4. What type of products are ideal for conditioning locks?
5. What is the difference between silky and yarn locks?
6. How is palm-rolling locksing carried out?
7. List the effects of wearing extensions over a long period of time.

Chapter 8 Shaving and face massage

Barbers are as popular now as ever with many more opening all the time, particularly in busy commercial areas where many men can pop out at lunchtime to have a quick haircut. Having the full works of a shave and a face massage is as indulgent for some men as a beauty spa is to some women and the demand is there for skilled barbers. Shaving with a cut-throat razor or designing a beard or moustache shape is a skill accomplished only by dedicated learners, but the finish is worthwhile. This chapter explores the methods, products and tools used for this art.

This chapter covers the following NVQ level 3 units:
H19 Provide shaving services
H20 Design and create a range of facial hair shapes
H34 Provide face massage services.

Shaving

Men's shaving and face massage is becoming more popular as today's clients need to look clean and well groomed. The art of shaving requires a steady hand, a great deal of skill and constant practice.

Shaving can be done either dry or wet. Dry shaving is done at home with electric razors, whereas in wet shaving the face is lathered and the hairs are removed when wet. Wet shaving is traditionally offered in salons where men's barbering takes place, and is becoming increasingly popular.

Safety

Using sharp razors in the salon is a risky process, so always follow health and safety legislation and local by-law procedures.

Local authority legislation

Local authorities around the country have different laws relating to the use of razors. Some areas will not allow the use of fixed-blade open razors and only disposable razors can be used.

TO DO

Find out through your local authority your responsibilities relating to the use of razors under the local by-laws and legislation.

TO DO

Re-read Chapter 1 regarding communication skills and answer the 'test your knowledge' questions.

Sharp razors must be kept closed and in a safe place (away from clients and children).

- Disposable razor blades must be safely disposed of (often by placing in a secure container, such as a wide-mouthed screw-topped bottle or a commercial 'sharps' container, before placing in the bin).

- Razors must be kept sterile (see Chapter 2) to prevent cross-infection if the client is accidentally cut (a small piece of cotton wool dipped in alum powder is needed to stop any bleeding). See Chapter 3 for what you should do if you accidentally cut yourself or your client.

Good communication is a vital part of shaving; you need to find out what your client requires.

- Does he want a **full** face shave?

- Does he want a **partial** face shave (does he want to keep his moustache or small beard)?

- Does he want an **outline** face shave (does he want the areas around his nape and sideburns shaved clean)?

- Would he like a **face massage** after the shave?

REMEMBER

If in doubt ask your supervisor. Re-read Chapter 1 for information on skin conditions.

Always consider:

- too much beard growth (more than 5 mm) will need to be removed before shaving. This will allow an easier shave.

- any unusual hair growth patterns, i.e. hair growing in lots of different directions

- any unusual facial features such as moles or birthmarks

- any adverse skin conditions such as an infection (e.g. folliculitis or impetigo), which would be spread and made worse by shaving and face massage (these should not be carried out)

- hot towels (a part of shaving) should not be used on a client with sensitive, chapped or blistered skin caused by heat or cold.

- facial piercings – you need to work carefully round these to avoid injury.

Tools and equipment

Barber's chair

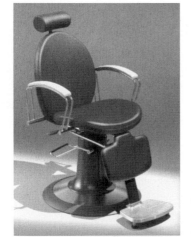

These are hydraulically controlled, and need to be locked at the correct height and position for you to work on the client comfortably. The chair is then reclined with the head rest inserted and locked in position so that the client is comfortably laid back in the chair ready for shaving.

Steamers

REMEMBER

Personal protective equipment – i.e. disposable protective gloves and protective workwear – should be worn during both shaving and face massage to prevent cross-infection through open cuts.

Hot towels are needed to soften and raise the facial hair and relax facial muscles before shaving. Towel steamers are used to hold hot towels ready for shaving, and are filled with water, which heats up to provide hot steamed towels. Always test the temperature of the hot towels gently on the client's skin, to make sure that they are not uncomfortably hot. If your salon does not have a steamer then the hot or cool towel can be prepared by following the diagrams below.

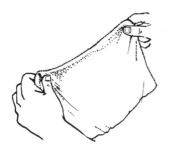

Folding a clean towel in half

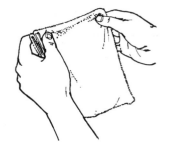

Folding towel in half again

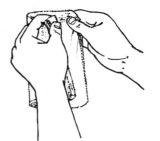

Getting ready to place towel under hot water

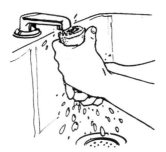

Saturating towel thoroughly with hot water

Lathering

Lathering the face removes dirt and helps to soften and lubricate the beard and hold the hair in an upright position. It also helps to provide a smooth, flat surface so that the razor can glide over the skin painlessly. Traditionally the lather was produced from soap and water. Nowadays foams, creams, gels or oils are used because they need little massaging and are more hygienic. They are applied with the tips of the fingers in an upward, circular motion. A shaving mug or bowl is filled with hot water. A clean, sterile shaving brush is then immersed, removed, and a small amount of foaming product is placed on the bristles. The brush is then rotated vigorously (like whisking an egg), either in the bowl of the shaving mug or in a second bowl, until lather is produced.

Gowns and towels

Men's gowns are usually fastened at the back for shaving. Shaving towels are often white, and smaller than normal hairdressing towels so that they fit comfortably around the face. Paper towels, tissue or shaving squares are also used for absorbing excess lather. Sponges are often used for very close shaving of dense beards to moisten and lubricate the skin. They must be kept clean and ideally kept for the sole use of that particular client.

Clippers

These may be used to partially remove a long, thick beard before shaving, in the same way that to restyle long hair to short the bulk of the hair is removed first.

Razors

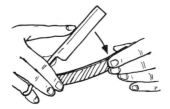

Opening razor safely

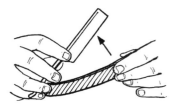

Closing razor safely

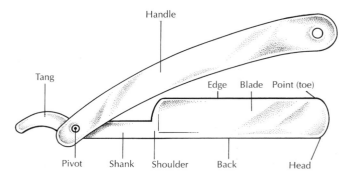

The parts of a razor

Safety razors with detachable blades

These are used without the guard for shaving and have disposable blades so that each client can have their own new sterile blade for each shave.

REMEMBER

● Hot towels are relaxing; they open the skin's pores and increase the blood flow to the skin surface.
● Cool towels are invigorating; they close the skin's pores, contract the skin and reduce the risk of infection, but not used before face massage as they contract the skin and muscles.

REMEMBER

Do not use tablet soap as it would be unhygienic to use the same soap on a large number of clients.

TO DO

Read Chapter 3 regarding the use of clippers for cutting facial hair.

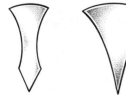

English/German hollow ground razor

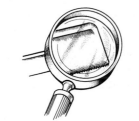

French solid razor

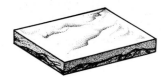

Magnified razor edge

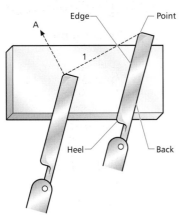

Belgian hone

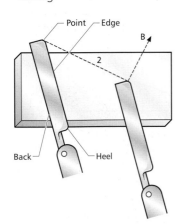

First position and stroke in honing

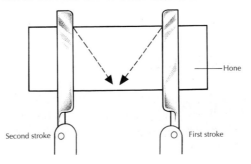

Second position and stroke in honing

Open razors

These have fixed blades and there are two types.

- **English/German hollow ground** – these are light, durable and pliable, but are too hard to use on sensitive skins.

- **French solid** – these are made from a softer metal and are more suitable for sensitive skins (and haircutting) but have to be sharpened more often.

Honing (or setting) fixed-blade razors

If you magnify the edge of a razor blade you can see very fine teeth at the edge (like a tiny saw).

When razors become blunt they have to be specially sharpened with a **hone** to create a new row of teeth and be able to cut hair again.

As razors lose their sharpness quite quickly, barbers have to hone (or sharpen) their razors themselves.

A hone is a rectangular block of quarried stone. The one most frequently used is a Belgian natural hone.

To hone a hollow-ground razor

- Wipe the surface of the hone to clean and free it from hair. Place it on a tissue.

- Lubricate the hone with fine oil.

- Stroke the razor blade diagonally across the hone, leading with the sharp cutting edge. Start with the heel and finish with the toe (point). Keep equal pressure on the blade, holding it flat as you complete the movement.

- Turn the razor on its back to commence the second stroke. Use your finger to turn the razor over (like rolling a pencil), not your wrist. As the razor is rolled over on its back, slide it upward towards the top corner of the same side. Now repeat the same diagonal movement.

- On completion, wipe the blade along the back with a tissue to clean it, close the blade, clean the hone and store both away safely.

To hone a French solid razor

- Clean and prepare the hone as before.

- Use a Belgian natural hone lubricated with a fine oil.

- The strokes should be shorter than those used for the hollow-ground razor, with only the razor edge resting, almost flat, on the hone. The stroke is more like a V shape with the razor turned on its back at the end of each stroke.

Honing a French solid razor

Testing the razor's edge

This is done by lightly pulling the razor across a moistened thumbnail.

- A perfectly sharp or keen edge will dig into the nail with a smooth, steady grip.
- A blunt edge will pull smoothly across the nail without any dragging or cutting.
- A nick in the razor will feel uneven when drawn across the nail.

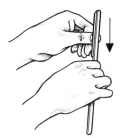

Testing sharpness of razor on moistened thumbnail

Stropping

A razor is stropped to preserve its cutting edge between honing and setting. Stropping cleans the razor's edge and realigns the teeth, creating a **whetted edge**.

Hanging strops are used for hollow-ground razors.

Solid strops are used for French solid razors.

New leather strops must be smeared with oil and left to soak overnight. The canvas side of the strop should be rubbed with soap. The following day both surfaces should be rubbed with a round glass bottle until a glazed surface appears.

REMEMBER

Always turn the razor on its back to avoid blunting or damaging the edge.

TO DO

Practise honing the razors available in your salon and ask your supervisor to comment on the results.

Stropping a hollow-ground razor

- Hang the strop on the hook then hold the free end with one hand and pull it horizontally out from the wall.
- Hold the razor in its straightened position with your other hand, keeping the razor shank between the first finger and thumb.
- Lie the razor flat and stroke it with the back first down the strop. When it has travelled two-thirds of the way down the strop, turn the razor on its back and repeat the stroke in the opposite direction.
- Although you will be slow to start with, your speed will increase with practice. Twelve strokes are usually sufficient to strop the razor.

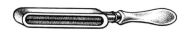

French or German strop

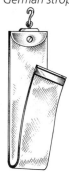

Leather and canvas strop

REMEMBER

Never turn the razor on its edge – you could cut and split the strop and damage the razor.

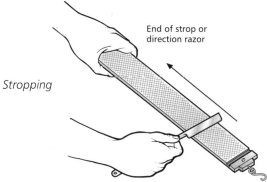

End of strop or direction razor

Stropping

First stroke

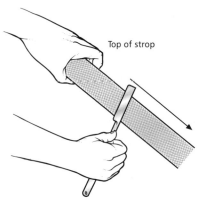

Top of strop

Second stroke

TO DO

- *Practise stropping the razors available in your salon. Ask your supervisor to comment on the results.*
- *Re-read Chapter 2 regarding the cleaning and sterilisation of all tools and equipment.*

Stropping a French solid razor

The movements are the same as before but the French strop is placed in a horizontal position on a work surface. The back of the razor is lifted slightly off the strop with edge of the blade resting flat and even on the strop. The same 12 strokes are needed.

Preparing the client

- Wash your hands and nails before starting. Keep your nails short for the face massage procedure.
- Ensure that your client's beard is clean and free from grease.
- Discuss with the client his requirements.
- Seat the gowned client in a reclined position with a clean paper towel placed over the head rest. Make sure the client is comfortable by adjusting the chair or gowns.
- Protect the client with a towel across his chest and tucked firmly into his neck.
- Check the face for any abnormalities, unusual beard growth patterns or adverse skin conditions.

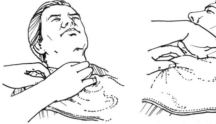

TO DO

- Re-read the section in Chapter 3 on gowning up, then watch a client being gowned up for a shave and a face massage in your salon Ask your supervisor what is the normal time allocation for this service.
- Read pages 154-155 regarding the preparation of equipment to check that you have not forgotten anything. For ease of use – keep your trolley on your right side if you are right-handed, left side if you are left-handed, avoiding any obstructions.

Lathering

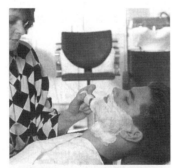

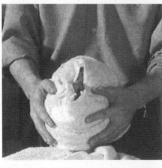

- Prepare the sterile steamed hot towel.
- Place the towel over the beard area, wrapping it over the face without covering the nose area so that the client can breathe easily.
- Strop the razor.
- Replace the cooled towel with a second hot towel.
- Prepare the brush and hot lather as previously described. Remove the second towel.
- Begin lathering the face by placing the brush on the tip of the chin and rotating it over the chin, cheeks and neck until all of the beard is covered with lather. To lather the upper lip the brush is spread by placing one finger in the centre of the bristles, preventing the lather from going up the client's nose or onto his lips.
- Keep the brush hot by dipping it into the hot water. The better the lather the easier the shave.

Shaving

Always carefully inspect the direction of the hair growth when shaving because the first-time-over shave is done in the same direction as the hair growth and the second-time-over shave is done against the direction of the hair growth (to cut the hair as closely as possible).

- It is essential that the angle of the razor and the direction of the razor hold are correct.
- The blade must be wiped clean to remove hair and lather between each razor stroke. Always wipe the razor on its back to prevent cutting your fingers.
- Use hot water for shaving – cold water will cause the razor to drag and be uncomfortable.

Holding the razor

There are two methods of holding the razor for shaving:
- forehand
- backhand.

You will need to practise both so that you can work at every angle of the face and neck.

First-time-over shave

The first-time-over shave is always done in the same direction as the hair growth – with the grain of the hair.

When you are stretching the skin for this shave, place your finger **behind** the razor instead of in front of it, as it is very difficult to get a firm grip on the skin when the face is slippery with lather.

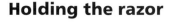

TO DO

- *Practise drawing the shaving movements on paper before working on a client.*
- *Once you have memorised these movements, secure an inflated balloon to practice your shaving techniques. Cover the balloon with shaving foam. The balloon will burst if you are holding the razor at an incorrect angle. Once you can remove the foam without difficulty, you are ready to try out your first shave.*
- *Ask your supervisor to comment on your techniques.*

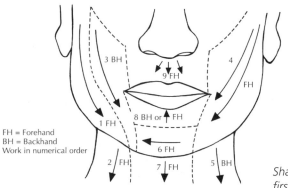

FH = Forehand
BH = Backhand
Work in numerical order

Shaving procedure: first-time-over

Method

- Wear your protective gloves.
- Hold the razor loosely with your thumb on the blade – the actual position will vary with the different strokes. Remember to dip the razor into the warm water.
- Begin the shave on the side nearest to you. Always start by holding the dry unlathered skin at the sideburn area to prevent your fingers slipping, pulling it taut when you start to shave.

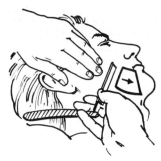

Backhand stroke

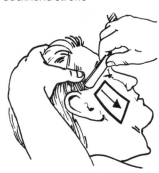

Forehand stroke

REMEMBER
- Always stretch the skin taut during shaving.
- This holds the hair up to the razor, allowing a closer cut.
- It also helps to prevent cuts to the skin.

REMEMBER
After each shaving stroke the razor blade needs to be cleaned of lather. Keep a paper towel or tissue nearby and wipe the back of the blade against the tissue to remove the lather without tearing the paper. Fold the tissue each time it is used.

REMEMBER
A right-handed barber should stand and start on the right-hand side; a left-handed one should stand and start on the left.

REMEMBER

Continual shaving on dark skin can cause the skin to become callous and make the skin darker in that area.

REMEMBER

Never shave tight-curly hair too close by shaving against the growth or grain – it is likely to cause ingrown hairs, creating swelling, infection, and possibly scarring.

REMEMBER

If you cut your client, a small piece of damp cotton wool dipped in alum powder should be applied to any cuts to the skin to stop the flow of blood. This is preferably applied by the client. Enter details into the accident book and remember to tell the relevant person.

- Move the razor in a slicing, scythe-like motion, following the movements shown in the diagram.
- Each side of the face should be completely shaved before starting the other, with the centre chin section left until last.
- Incorporate each side of the upper lip area when shaving that side of the face, leaving just the centre section which is then shaved downwards while gently pressing the tip of the nose upwards to tighten the skin.
- When one side of the face has been completed, turn the client's head towards you to make it easier to shave the other side.
- To shave the point of the chin, pull the skin tight between the finger and thumb, then use the middle of the razor blade to shave across the chin.
- Finish by shaving the neck downwards.

Second-time-over shave

This shave is important because it ensures that the hair is cut as closely as possible giving a clean finished result. The hair is cut in an upward movement **against the growth**.

This is usually the final shave unless the client is very dark haired with a strong beard growth. When this is the case, it is followed by a sponge shave, which entails soaking a small sponge in hot water then dragging it across the face, closely followed by the razor.

Method

- Re-lather the face.
- Start the shave at the collar area, using your fingers to hold the dry, unlathered skin.
- Move upwards in backhand strokes, completing one side of the face before starting the other (as in the diagram).

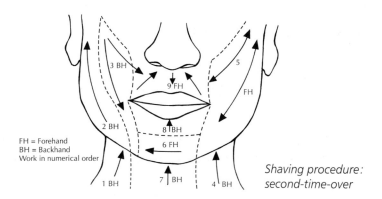

FH = Forehand
BH = Backhand
Work in numerical order

Shaving procedure: second-time-over

- Clean the face with a damp, warm towel or sponge, then pat dry gently with another clean towel.
- Apply a small amount of talcum powder to make sure that the skin is thoroughly dry.
- Finish with an after-shave lotion, which is an astringent and will close the pores, leaving the skin feeling fresh and clean.
- Sit the client in an upright position and check that he is satisfied with the result.

Always check beforehand with your supervisor that you have chosen the proper correction to match the fault

Fault	Cause	Correction
Client discomfort	Wrong positioning	Adjust either the chair setting or the gowns and towels
	Towels too hot	Replace hot towel with a cooler one
Uneven shave	Blunt razor	Resharpen the razor's edge
	Incorrect skin tension	Stretch the skin smoothly
	Incorrect razor angle	Recorrect the angle to remove the hair
	Poor lathering	Re-lather evenly
Painful razoring	Shaving dry	Relubricate the skin with lather
	Blunt razor	Test the edge and hone if necessary
	Razoring squarely	Recorrect and adjust the razor angle
Facial cuts	Insufficient skin tension	Stretch the skin taut
	Blunt razor blade	Test the edge, resharpen by honing
	Heavy razoring	Hold the razor more lightly
	Incorrect razor angle	Adjust the angle of the razor
Skin rashes caused by irritation	Shaving dry	Relubricate the skin with lather
	Razor drag	Recorrect and adjust the razor angle
	Razor blunt	Test the edge, hone and strop
	Razoring against the natural growth	Razor with the growth
	Shaving too close	Let the skin rest
	Lather drying out	Keep moist, check your speed
	Towels too hot	Check and cool
Ingrowing hairs	Continually shaving curly hair too close	Avoid shaving too close
	Building up of skin cells	Exfoliate regularly

Cutting men's facial hair

Men's facial hair can enhance the wearer's appearance by apparently altering the shape of the face – it can make a long face appear narrower, or completely disguise a receding chin.

Fashions and trends in beards, moustaches and sideburns change rapidly, although some cultures, such as Sikhs and Orthodox Jews, have very strict rules as to how facial hair should be worn.

Here are some examples of the many different types that have been worn in the past and some that are still worn today.

| Medium full beard | Balbo beard | Goatee beard | Handlebar and chin puff |

REMEMBER

A man has to consciously grow a beard. He is making a statement about himself – so cutting facial hair is just as important as cutting scalp hair.
Before you begin to cut, consider your client's reasons for wearing facial hair.

TO DO

● Research the latest magazines and journals for illustrations of **current** beard and moustache shapes.
● Add these to your style book.

Spade or Shenandoah beard

Old Dutch beard

Hulihee beard

Franz Josef beard

Chin curtain beard

Pencil line moustache

Handlebar moustache

Howie moustache

Square button, Hitler or Charlie Chaplin moustache

Walrus or Old Bill moustache

Adolph Menjou moustache

The major

The general

Shermanic moustache

Painter's brush moustache

The military

Walrus moustache

TO DO

Check with your supervisor to see if your salon has any particular requirements for gowning up when cutting men's facial hair.

TO DO

Re-read about client consultation in Chapter 1, complete your consultation sheet and confirm the beard/moustache shape with the client by the use of photographs. Check the outcome of your consultation with your supervisor.

TO DO

● Re-read Chapter 1 regarding abnormal hair and scalp conditions.
● List and describe the effects of dealing with the non-infectious and infectious skin conditions that must be considered before cutting facial hair.

Head and face shapes

- The **oval** face shape is ideal and suits any style.
- For **round** and **square** face shapes beards need to be styled to reduce the width and to be cut flatter at the sides.
- The **long** face shape needs to be made to appear shorter and wider. A moustache will help this.
- A beard will help to cover and minimise a small or **receding chin**.
- Sideburns may be part of the facial or scalp hair, or blend with both.

Natural growth patterns

Facial hair grows in certain directions in the same way that scalp hair does. It mostly grows downwards and outwards, and occasionally grows in circular shapes under the chin.

Hair structures and textures

Examine the hair carefully – it may be straight or curly, coarse or fine, dense or sparse and will need cutting accordingly. Facial or beard hair is generally wavy or curly and much stronger and coarser than scalp hair.

- Look at the distribution of the facial hair – there may be too much, e.g. a great deal of hair on the neck area which needs to be removed.
- Or there may be too little – e.g. a scarred area or facial alopecia having no hair growth that cannot be seen until it is cut short (then it is too late!).

Preparation

Gowning up

The client's clothes must be protected as normal, and both of his eyes need to be covered with a feathered-out strip of neck wool.

A towel should be placed diagonally across the client's chest and one side tucked into the collar. The opposite corner of the towel is then folded diagonally over the top and tucked into the other side of the collar. There should be no gap between the client's neck and the towel.

The outline shape of the facial hair must be perfectly balanced and symmetrical when complete. It is sometimes difficult to see this shape if the background is the same colour as his hair. Therefore try to use a light-coloured gown or towel for dark beards, and darker gowns or towels for lighter beards.

Positioning your client

You will need to work with your client in a reclined position by adjusting the barber's chair and head rest. (If you don't have a barber's chair recline the client at the back wash-basin and place a towel under his neck for comfort.)

Cutting tools

The tools used for cutting moustaches and beards are often lighter and smaller than usual. This is for precision and accuracy when you are working with delicate shapes and patterns in small areas.

Disentangling

Disentangle the beard by combing it downwards with a wide-toothed comb.

Cutting methods

Scissor over comb

Using small sections, start in the centre of the chin and work out towards the right side and then the left side. Always keep the comb and scissors moving. The closer your comb is held to the face the shorter the cut will be.

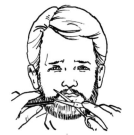
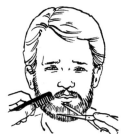
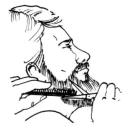
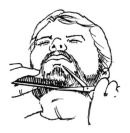

Trimming moustache and beard   *Retouch work*   *Trimming excess hair*   *Tapering and blending the beard*

Clipper over comb

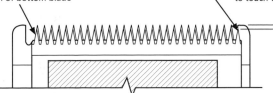

Extreme left-hand tooth of top blade must be covering, or be to the left of, the first small tooth of bottom blade

Extreme right-hand tooth of top blade must be touching the big tooth on the bottom blade

End of top blade teeth should be 1/32" to 1/16", 0.79 mm to 1.59 mm, back from bottom blade. This is important so that the clipper doesn't cut too close or allow the moving blade to touch the skin

Cordless or rechargeable clippers are much easier to use for facial hair, because you are continually twisting and turning the clippers during cutting. Clipper guards are useful for short beards but may become entangled in longer ones. The final shape may be outlined with clippers.

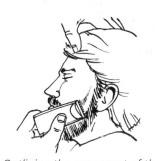

Outlining the upper part of the beard freehand, using clippers

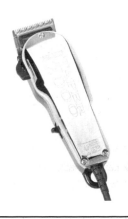

Clippers with adjustable blades have a lever or a switch which will either increase or decrease the space between the moving and still-cutting blades. The smaller the gap between the blades the closer the cut will be to the skin.

Clippers must be kept clean from hair cuttings and regularly oiled with professional clipper oil. Clipper oil is a very thin natural oil which does not evaporate or slow down the power of the clippers. A few drops must be placed between the blades, every few haircuts.

To clean the blades thoroughly you need to loosen the screws beneath the blades to free them. Loose cut hairs can then be brushed out and cleaned away.

When you put the blades back together you must realign them so that they don't cut too close or allow the moving blade to touch the skin.

Freehand cutting

The outlines of beards or moustaches are usually done freehand, without holding the hair in place with a comb or your fingers. Always support your scissors with your first finger when cutting a moustache to protect the client's lips.

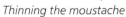

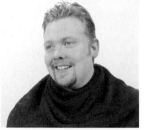
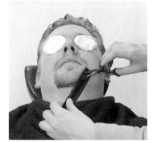
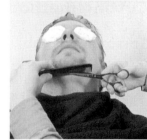

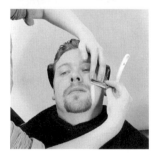
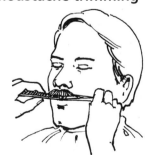
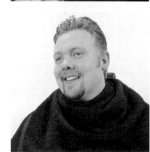

Moustache trimming

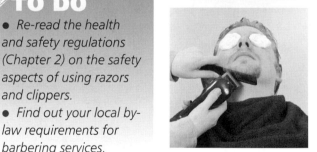

Thinning the moustache   *Trimming the moustache*   *Shaving unwanted part of beard*

Razoring

A disposable open razor can be used in the same way as lining out to remove any unwanted hair outside the desired shape.

TO DO

Check with your supervisor and find out how long it should take you to:
- cut a beard
- cut a moustache.

TO DO

- Re-read the health and safety regulations (Chapter 2) on the safety aspects of using razors and clippers.
- Find out your local by-law requirements for barbering services.

REMEMBER

After cutting it is important to exfoliate around the hair outline to soften the skin and prevent ingrowing hair. Suitable products include:
- Facial scrubs
- Exfoliating masks
- Fruit acid peels.

Finishing off

Remove all the beard clippings from your client with your neck brush then ask the client if he is satisfied with the result as you show him in the mirror.

TO DO

Read Chapter 9, Indian head massage, for information on bones and muscles of the face, lymphatic system and skin ageing.

REMEMBER

Accidents can happen – re-read Chapter 3 regarding cutting yourself or the client in the salon. You are more likely to cut the client during barbering than when you are working on a female client. Use alum powder on a small piece of damp cotton wool to stop any bleeding, and ask the client to hold it on to the cut.

TEST YOUR KNOWLEDGE

1 Why is it important to match beard shapes with the client's facial characteristics?

2 Why is it important to consult with your client before cutting his facial hair?

3 Describe the health and safety requirements regarding the use of cutting equipment.

4 Describe the difference between adjusting and aligning clippers.

5 Describe your responsibilities under the Electricity at Work Regulations 1992.

6 What should you do if you accidentally cut your own skin?

7 What should you do if you accidentally cut your client's skin?

8 What particular safety considerations must be taken into account when cutting facial hair?

9 How should you dispose of used razor blades?

10 How should you prepare a fixed-blade open razor for use?

11 Why should the skin be stretched taut during shaving?

12 Describe six problems that may occur during shaving, their causes, and how to correct them.

13 Why should you seek the advice of your supervisor when you are unsure of how to correct any mistakes?

14 Name two finishing products that may be used after shaving and describe their uses.

15 Why is it important to consult with the client throughout the shaving process?

Face massage

Massage is usually carried out after shaving to aid skin elasticity, tone the facial muscles and encourage the removal of toxins. The main benefit of a face massage is to relax the client.

TO DO

Re-read Chapter 1 to remind yourself of the functions and make-up of the skin.

Make sure that you confirm the desired finished result with the client before you start work, particularly regarding the choice of finishing products to be used.

Before starting the massage, make sure that the client's hair and clothing are well protected from the massage cream. Prepare the equipment and make sure that your hands and nails are clean, and wear protective gloves.

Check the client's skin for any facial piercings, cuts or abrasions, bruises, moles or adverse skin conditions.

REMEMBER

Be prepared!
It is better to be practised and competent with new products and materials beforehand rather than have to turn clients away.

REMEMBER

Health and safety – never contaminate products by dipping your fingers into pots and jars. Always use a spatula, and place the product onto the back of your hand, closing the container immediately after use. Applicators are the most hygienic to use.

Method

- Steam the face with two hot towels.
- Apply the massage cream lightly over the face with stroking, spreading **effleurage** movements.
- Stroke fingers across the forehead with up and down movements.
- Manipulate your fingers across the forehead with a circular **pétrissage** movement.

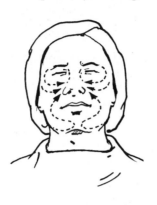 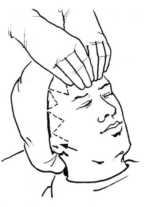 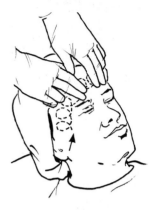

Applying cleansing cream lightly over the face with effleurage stroking, spreading and circular movements

Stroke fingers across forehead with up and down movements

Use petrissage across forehead with a circular movement

- Stroke your fingers upwards along the side of the nose.
- Apply a circular movement over the side of the nose and use a light, stroking movement around the eyes.
- Manipulate the temples with a wide circular movement. Also manipulate the front and back of the ears with a circular **pétrissage** movement.

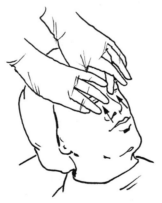 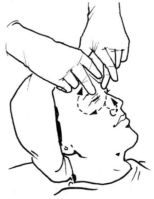 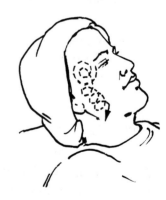

Stroke fingers upwards along the side of the nose

Apply a circular movement over side of nose and use a light, stroking movement around the eyes

Manipulate the temples with petrissage circular movement. Also manipulate the front and back of the ears with a circular movement

- Gently stroke both of your thumbs across the upper lip.
- Use a circular movement from the corners of the mouth, working up to the cheeks and temples, and again working along the lower jawbone from the tip of the chin to the ear.

- Stroke your fingers with an **effleurage** movement from under the chin and neck to the back of the ears and up towards the temples.

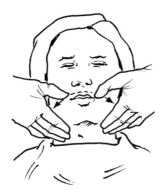

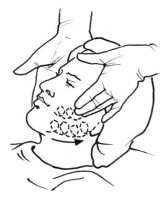

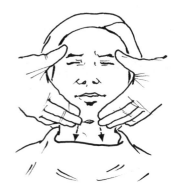

Gently stroke both thumbs across upper lip

Use a circular movement to manipulate around the jaw

Manipulate fingers from under chin and neck to back of ears and up to temples

- Complete the treatment with another hot towel followed by a cool towel. An astringent may be used to close the pores and tighten up the skin.

Finishing products

The range of men's facial products have increased considerably in the past few years and you, the professional, must be able to advise your client on the best and most suitable products to use.

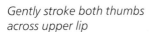

TO DO

- *Visit your local wholesalers and manufacturers to find out what men's products are available.*
- *Ask clients about the skincare ranges they use and build up a file of information.*

Some clients purchase such products because they enjoy the pleasant perfume; others prefer unperfumed products. Many manufacturers supply 'testers' so that clients can choose the perfume they prefer.

- Talcum powder may be used to soothe and dry the skin, helping to reduce the effect of oily, shiny skin.
- Face creams will soothe and moisturise and help to correct dry skin conditions.
- Aftershave lotions will close the skin's pores and reduce both skin irritation and the risk of infection. They act both as an astringent and a mild antiseptic, leaving a pleasant smell.
- Aftershave balms will soothe the skin as they contain conditioners and leave a pleasant smell. They do not sting, unlike after-shave lotions.

Vibro massage

This is a mechanical massage that can be used instead of a hand massage. It produces very strong **tapotement** (tapping) movements, which are suitable only for fleshy areas of skin. It can be very uncomfortable for the client when used on bony areas such as the forehead and jawline, and it must **never** be used around the eyes or on the nose.

REMEMBER

Use the vibro gently and carefully. If it feels too strong for the client then use the attachments over your hand.

Use the vibro in the same order and in the same direction as in the diagrams for the hand massage (see page 166).

Sit the client upright and check that he is satisfied with the result.

MASSAGE – MOVEMENT	EFFECT
Effleurage – stroking	Soothing and relaxing
Pétrissage – deep kneading	Stimulates muscles and nerves, improving the circulation
Tapotement – tapping	Tones the muscles, breaks down fatty deposits and increases the blood flow to the skin
Vibro massage – mechanical tapping	Tones the muscles, breaks down fatty deposits and increases the blood flow to the skin

TO DO

- Read Chapter 2 regarding keeping your work area clean and tidy, and dispose of waste materials.
- Ask your supervisor if these are the procedures used in your salon.

TEST YOUR KNOWLEDGE

1 Describe the health and safety requirements that should be considered and taken into account during shaving and massaging.

2 When would you not carry out shaving and face massage?

3 Why should you prepare and position your tools and equipment properly before commencing a shave or face massage?

4 Describe how hot and cool towels are used and the effects they have on the skin.

5 Name and describe each type of face massage technique.

6 Why is it important to report both product stock and sundry shortages to the relevant person?

7 Why is it important to keep your work area clean and tidy, dispose of waste materials and avoid cross-infections and infestations?

Chapter 9 Indian head massage

The skill of Indian head massage can be used anywhere in hairdressing and barbering salons and is an added service that is becoming more popular, with many practitioners qualifying each year. If done properly this massage can be as beneficial to the giver as it is to the receiver. The skills of the massage should be followed closely to gain the most benefit and this chapter aims to cover all the aspects of this fantastic service. The material in this chapter has been used by permission of Francesca Gould.

This chapter covers the following NVQ level 3 unit:
BT20 Indian head massage.

What is Indian head massage?

Indian head massage is an ancient practice based on the Ayurvedic healing system in India. Ayurvedic medicine is a holistic healing system, which combines natural therapies and encompasses the mind, body and spirit. It strives to restore balance and inner harmony to the mind, body and spirit to improve the health of the individual by balancing the chakras and rebalancing the body's energy systems through diet, exercise and meditation.

Indian head massage is often practised in the home. Traditionally, as the hot climate of India is very drying, oils are used to keep the hair shiny and in good condition.

The skill is handed down through the generations with children being taught from the age of six. Mothers will massage their babies every day until the age of three, and up until the age of six children receive a massage once or twice a week.

Indian head massage can help relax, soothe or invigorate the receiver. Using their hands, the therapist kneads, rubs and squeezes the body's soft tissues.

Indian head massage treatment is becoming very popular in the West because it has advantages over other massage treatments, as it fits well into busy people's lives.

The massage can be carried out almost anywhere while the client is still wearing their clothes – you may have seen Indian head massages being offered on a chair in the street during summer months. It is quick, little equipment is needed and it can be done with or without creams or oils.

The body

Before a massage can be carried out successfully the therapist should understand the areas of the body they are working on. During Indian head massage treatment these areas are:

1   Head
2   Neck
3   Shoulders
4   Upper back
5   Arms
6   Hands

The skeleton

The bone is living tissue and is constantly renewing itself. It is the hardest of all connective tissue in the body and is made up of 30% living tissue and 70% minerals and water.

Function of bones

The skeleton is the framework of the body. It gives the body its shape and supports the weight of all the other tissues. The bones protect vital organs from injury. Blood cells are produced within the marrow of some bones in the body. Bones store minerals, mainly calcium and phosphorous. If these minerals are needed elsewhere in the body the bones release them into the bloodstream.

Bones of the upper body

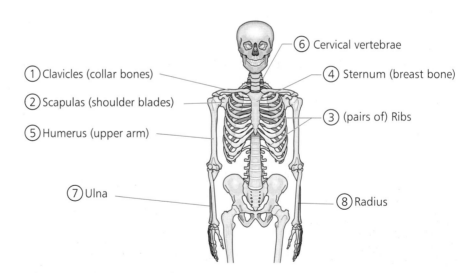

Bones of the upper body

1   2 Clavicles – collar bones
2   2 Scapulas – shoulder blades
3   12 pairs of ribs
4   1 Sternum – breast bone
5   1 Humerus – upper arm
6   7 Cervical vertebrae – in the neck
7   1 Ulna – forearm
8   1 Radius – forearm

Bones of the skull and face

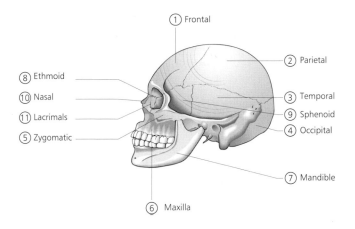
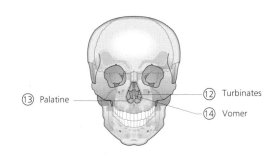

Bones of the skull and face

1   1 Frontal – forehead
2   2 Parietal – two bones on the sides and top
3   2 Temporal – two bones at the sides under the parietals
4   1 Occipital – back of the skull
5   2 Zygomatic – cheekbones
6   1 Maxilla – upper jaw
7   1 Mandible – lower jaw (the only moveable bone in the skull)
8   1 Ethmoid – eye socket and nasal cavities
9   1 Sphenoid – helps to form the base of the skull
10   2 Nasal – bridge of the nose
11   2 Lacrimals – eye sockets
12   3 Turbinates – nasal cavity
13   2 Palatine – L-shaped bones form the walls of the nasal cavity and part of the roof of the mouth.
14   1 Vomer – back of the mouth up towards the nasal septum

Bones of the hand

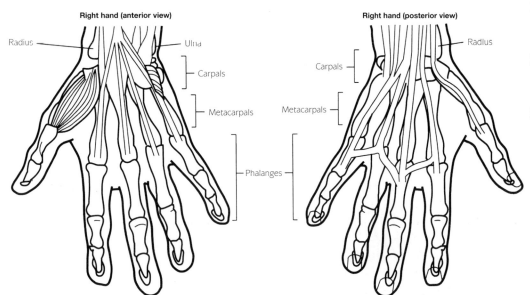

1   Metacarpals – between the carpals and middle knuckle
2   Phalanges – finger bones from the middle knuckle to the fingertip
3   Carpals – collective word for the bones in the palm of the hand. From left to right looking at the back of a left hand nearest to fingers first.

Muscles

Muscles are formed from bundles of long fibres, which are made up of threadlike **myofibrils**. The myofibrils in turn are made of **filaments**. These filaments move in and out of the myofibrils when the muscle contracts and relaxes rather like a telescopic pole. The muscle fibres are covered with a 'skin' called **fascia**.

Muscle tone

Muscles are never completely relaxed. Imagine standing very still; even though you are not 'moving a muscle' most of the muscles in your body are partially contracted. If all your muscles relaxed you would fall to the floor. This is called muscle tone. Muscle tone varies throughout the body depending on how you are standing or sitting, as these positions will use some muscles more or less than others.

Back, shoulders and arms

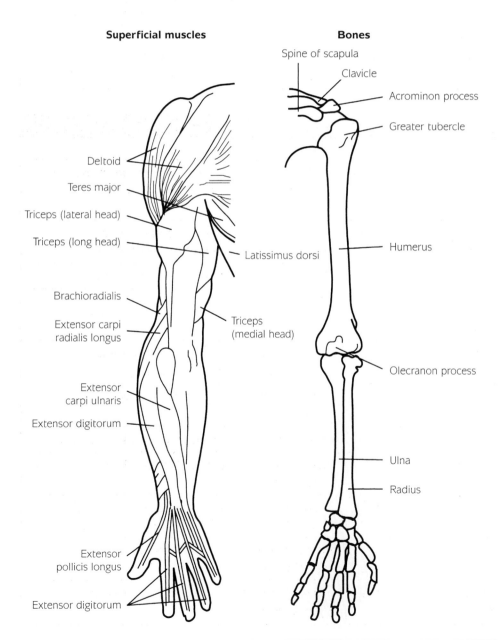

Superficial muscles

Deltoid
Teres major
Triceps (lateral head)
Triceps (long head)
Brachioradialis
Extensor carpi radialis longus
Extensor carpi ulnaris
Extensor digitorum
Extensor pollicis longus
Extensor digitorum
Latissimus dorsi
Triceps (medial head)

Bones

Spine of scapula
Clavicle
Acrominon process
Greater tubercle
Humerus
Olecranon process
Ulna
Radius

1 Biceps – front of upper arm – flexes the forearm
2 Triceps – back of upper arm – extends the forearm
3 Brachialis – above the elbow – flexes the forearm
4 Extensors and flexors – lower arm – moves the wrist
5 Deltoid – shoulder – for full arm movement
6 Radialis trapezius – top of the back and neck – lifts the shoulders and draws the head backwards
7 Erector spinae – both sides of the vertebrae – back movement and holding the body upright.

MUSCLES OF THE UPPER BODY

Muscle	Position	Origin	Insertion	Action
1 Biceps brachii	Down anterior surface of the humerus	Scapula	Radius and flexor muscles in forearm	Flexes the forearm
2 Triceps	Posterior surface of the humerus	Humerus and scapula	Ulna	Extends the forearm
3 Brachialis	On the anterior aspect of humerus beneath the biceps	Humerus	Ulna	Flexes the forearm
4 Extensors and flexors	Lower arm	Humerus	Ulna	Move the wrist
5 Deltoid	A thick, triangular muscle that caps the shoulder	Clavicle and scapula	Humerus	Abducts the arm and draws it backwards and forwards
6 Radialis trapezius	Forms a large, kite-shaped muscle across the top of the back and neck	Occipital bone and vertebrae	Scapula and clavicle	Lifts the clavicle as in shrugging and also draws the head backwards
7 Erector spinae	Three groups of muscles found on either side of vertebrae	Vertebrae, ribs, iliac crest	Cervical and lumbar vertebrae, ribs	Extends the spine and so helps to hold the body in an upright position

Head, face and neck

MUSCLES OF THE HEAD, FACE AND NECK

Muscle	Position	Action
1 Sterno-cleidomastoid	Runs from the top of the sternum to the clavicle and temporal bones	Both together bend head forward; one muscle only rotates the head and draws it towards the opposite shoulder
2 Platysma	Extends from the lower jaw to the chest and covers the front of the neck	Depresses lower jaw and draws lower lip outwards and draws up the skin of the chest
3 Occipito-frontalis	Across the forehead	Draws scalp forward and raises eyebrows
4 Orbicularis oculi	Around the eyes	Closes the eye
5 Zygomaticus minor	Along the upper lip	Lifts the upper lip
6 Zygomaticus major	Extends diagonally from the corners of the mouth	Lifts the corners of the mouth upwards and outwards, as in smiling or laughing
7 Risorius	Extends diagonally from either side of the mouth	Draws the corner of the mouth outwards, as in grinning
8 Mentalis	On the chin	Raises and protrudes lower lip, wrinkles skin of chin
9 Orbicularis oris	Surrounds the mouth	Closure and protrusion of the lips, changes shape of lips for speech
10 Buccinator	In each cheek, to the side of the mouth	Compresses cheeks, as in whistling and blowing, and draws the corners of the mouth in, as in sucking
11 Masseter	The cheeks	The muscle of chewing: it closes the mouth and clenches the teeth
12 Temporalis	Extends from the temple region to the upper jaw bone	Raises the lower jaw and draws it backwards, as in chewing

The effect of massage on the muscles

- The blood supply to the muscle is increased during massage bringing fresh oxygen and nutrients and removing waste products such as lactic acid, so massage can help to alleviate muscle fatigue. The muscle is warmed because of the increased blood flow and, because warm muscles contract more efficiently than when cold, the likelihood of injury is reduced.

- Massage helps to relieve pain, stiffness and fatigue in muscles as the waste products are removed and normal functioning is quickly restored. The increased oxygen and nutrients aid tissue repair and recovery of the muscle.

- Massage can help the breakdown of **fibrositic nodules**, also termed knots, that develop within a muscle because of tension, injuries or poor posture. They are commonly found in the shoulder area.

- Massage helps to increase the tone of the muscles and delays wasting away of muscles through lack of use. There is also a decrease of muscle tone with ageing.

The skin

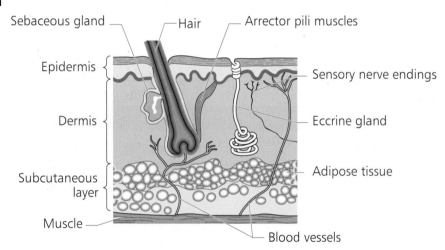

The effects of ageing on the skin

As the skin's elasticity decreases, character lines are formed together with fine lines and wrinkles. The skin becomes more permeable leading to dehydration and the pores become more open. There is a decrease in both sebum production and activity of the sudiferous glands. As the cellular regeneration slows down, the skin becomes thinner around the eyes and there is an increase in hyper-pigmentation. There is also an accelerated growth of fine lanugo hair.

Effect of massage on the skin

- The circulation is improved and so fresh blood brings nutrients to the sebaceous glands; therefore sebum production is increased. More sebum helps to make the skin soft and supple.

- The sweat glands become more active and so more sweat is excreted. Toxins such as urea and other waste products are eliminated from the body in this way.

- Massage also causes the top layer of dead skin cells to be shed (desquamation), which improves the condition of the skin, giving it a healthy glow.

- The sensory nerve endings can either be soothed or stimulated, depending on the massage movements used.

- When massage and essential oils are used together the skin's health and appearance can be greatly improved.

ADVANCED HAIRDRESSING

Effects of environmental and lifestyle factors on the skin

Stress:

- May cause the skin to appear dull and sallow
- May cause premature ageing.

Smoking:

- Reduces the amount of oxygen reaching the skin and results in both dryness and the dilating of the capillaries
- Causes the formation of premature lines around the lips.

Diet:

- The skin becomes dehydrated due to lack of fluid
- Poor diet can cause skin allergies and disorders
- Alcohol dehydrates the skin and deprives it of vitamin reserves
- Caffeine prevents the absorption of vitamins and minerals and the skin appears unhealthy.

Climate:

- Ultraviolet light can contribute to premature ageing of the skin
- Extreme temperature can lead to the formation of broken capillaries
- In hot, dry climates the skin becomes dehydrated due to water loss
- Less sebum is produced in cold climates, reducing the skin's protection and allowing moisture to evaporate.

Lymph

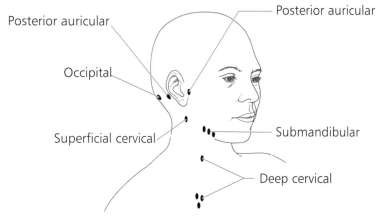

Lymph glands of the head and neck

There are approximately 600 lymph nodes scattered around the body. Lymph nodes filter out harmful substances from the lymph such as bacteria. Lymphocytes and monocytes in the nodes destroy this harmful bacteria. The glands which swell more noticeably in the neck when you are unwell are lymph nodes frantically producing antibodies.

Effects of massage on lymph

Massage helps to stimulate the flow of lymph and strokes should be directed towards the nearest set of lymph nodes. Massage will help to drain away excess fluid and will help prevent fluid retention.

Effects of massage on blood flow

Massage pushes the blood through the veins speeding up their progress around the body. Stroking (**effleurage**) movements toward the heart will help return the blood back to the heart so fresh oxygenated blood will be released into the veins and arteries and so will nourish the tissues and help with tissue repair.

The nervous system

The brain and the spinal cord form the central nervous system. Nerves carry electrical impulses from the central nervous system to all parts of the body. The autonomic-nerve impulses make muscles contract, or glands produce enzymes or hormones.

The nerves also carry impulses back to the central nervous system from the sense organs of the body, such as the eyes, ears or skin. These impulses make us aware of the changes in our surroundings or in ourselves. The nerves which connect the body to the central nervous system make up the peripheral nervous system.

Chakras

The Indian head massage routine includes chakra balancing work. The body has seven major chakras: crown, brow (third eye), throat, heart, solar plexus, hara (sacrum) and base (root). An important part of Indian head massage is working with the higher chakras, the crown (*sahasrara*), third eye (*ajna*) and throat (*vishuddha*). Minor chakras are also found in the feet, on the palms of the hands and at joints.

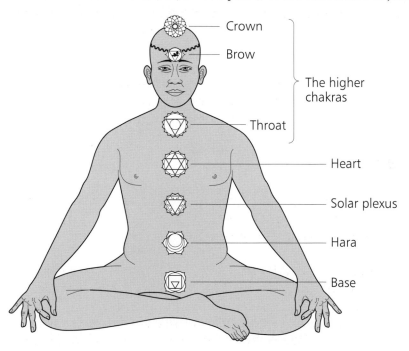

The chakras

The chakras are centres of energy that are located about 2.5 cm (an inch) away from the body and should ideally spin in a clockwise direction. Each chakra resembles a flower and its petals represent energy channels through which energy passes. Each chakra has a different number of petals. The energy (prana) for the chakras is supplied from the universe. Prana is an Indian word meaning 'life-force energy'. It enters the body through these energy centres. To ensure health, all the chakras need to be open, unblocked and in balance with each other.

Higher chakras

The crown chakra is called the master chakra and can help to open up and balance the six other chakras of the body. It is important that this chakra is not blocked, otherwise energy will not be able to run freely from all the other chakras to it.

Working with this chakra will cause energy to be sent to where it is needed in the body and so promote healing. The crown chakra is the place through which the universe sends its energy into the body.

Marma points

The Marmas (vital points) are a very important part of Ayurvedic anatomy and surgery. A Marma point is defined as an anatomical site where flesh, veins, arteries, tendons, bones and joints meet up. There are 107 Marma points throughout the body, of which 37 are in the treatment area. Each point has its own intelligence and consciousness, which co-ordinate with the mind and body. This ancient form of treatment dating back to between 1500–1200 BC involves using the fingers to stimulate the Marma points, thereby promoting physical and mental rehabilitation. As with acupuncture, these points correspond to internal organs and systems of the body which react to manual stimulation.

There are wide applications for Marma massage. Stroke victims benefit from the treatment, which can clear away obstructions which delay information being communicated between the muscles, nerves and the brain. This helps the brain to 're-learn' how to control and co-ordinate the muscles and nerves after illness or injury.

It generally takes 2–6 sessions to restore the body to health depending on the individual's damage to body and mind. In the case of stroke victims weekly treatments should be carried out over 3–6 months.

Consultation

The consultation process for Indian head massage, as with all specialist massages, is vitally important. A professional consultation should take around 15 minutes and a consultation form should be filled in by the client.

During the consultation, you should establish if there are any medical reasons why the treatment should not go ahead, such as high blood pressure, recent head or neck injury, epilepsy or migraine. These and more contraindications are given in more detail later in the chapter. You can both decide which, if any, oils are to be used, what the client's expectations are, whether they want you to concentrate on an aching shoulder or just want overall relaxation.

Indian head massage is a holistic treatment, which means that we take into account the mind, body and spirit to improve the health of an individual. This is why during the consultation you should ask about lifestyle factors including hobbies and stress levels. You can give the client advice regarding their lifestyle that will help relieve stress, tiredness and persistent aches and pains, such as taking up yoga and tai chi.

TO DO

Look at the consultation forms available in your salon. Read through the questions carefully to familiarise yourself with it and ask your supervisor if there is anything you do not understand.

INDIAN HEAD MASSAGE CONSULTATION FORM

NAME: .... TEL NO: ....
ADDRESS: ....

EMAIL ADDRESS: ....
D.O.B: .... OCCUPATION: ....

MEDICAL QUESTIONNAIRE
Do you suffer with or have you suffered with any of the following:
Any recent head or neck injury? ....
Severe brusing on area being treated? ....
Epilepsy? ....
Recent haemorrhage? ....
High or low blood pressure? ....
Migraines? ....
Thrombosis or embolism? ....
Diabetes? ....
Spastic conditions? ....
Dysfunction of the nervous system? ....
Skin disorders? ....
Scalp infections? ....
Cuts or abrasions in area being treated? ....
A recent operation? ....
....

Are you pregnant? ....
Are you currently taking any medication? ....
Is GP referral required? .... Yes/No ....
Name of doctor: ....
Surgery address: .... Tel no: ....

LIFESTYLE

Do you drink alcohol? If so how often? ....
Do you smoke? If so how many each day? ....
Would you say your stress levels are: high/average/low? ....
Details if levels are high: ....
Would you say your energy levels are: high/average/poor? ....
What are your hobbies? How do you relax? ....
....

Why have you come for an Indian head massage treatment? ....
....

Additional notes: ....
....

Client declaration
The information I have given regarding my medical details is accurate. I will promptly notify the therapist of any future changes to my health.

Client signature: .... Date: ....

Date: ....
Oils used: ....
Areas of tension: ....
Comments: ....
....

Contraindications to massage

Indian head massage is a very safe treatment. However, there are certain conditions that the therapist should be aware of which may prevent treatment being carried out or require the advice of a doctor.

The contraindications to Indian head massage include:
- any recent head or neck injury
- severe bruising, cuts or abrasions in the treatment area
- epilepsy
- recent haemorrhage
- high blood pressure
- low blood pressure
- migraine
- history of thrombosis or embolism
- diabetes
- spastic conditions
- dysfunction of the nervous system
- skin disorders/scalp infections
- recent operations.

Massage movements

While carrying out the Indian head massage routine you will use different types of massage movements called effleurage, pétrissage, tapotement, vibrations and frictions.

Effleurage

Effleurage (a French word meaning 'stroking') always begins and ends the massage on each area. It is also usually performed after tapotement massage movements to soothe the area. The effleurage movement can be superficial (using light pressure) or deep, using slightly deeper pressure. These movements must always follow the direction of venous return (blood in the veins) back to the heart and also in the direction of lymphatic drainage towards a group of lymph nodes. The hands stay in contact with the body during the return stroke.

Uses of effleurage
- To distribute the massage medium so that the whole area is lubricated
- To introduce the therapist's hands
- To warm up the area so deeper massage movements can be used
- To link massage movements together, so that the massage flows
- To relax the receiver.

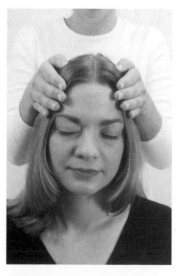

Effleurage movement

Effect of effleurage

- Improves the blood and lymphatic circulation
- Aids desquamation (removal of dead skin cells) so the skin will look healthier and feel smoother
- Soothes nerve endings, thus inducing relaxation.

Pétrissage

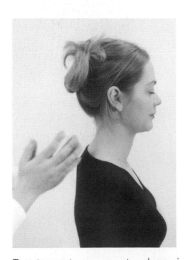

Pétrissage movement

Pétrissage (a French word meaning 'kneading') movements are deeper movements in which soft tissues are compressed. These movements either press the muscle on to the bone or lift it away from the bone. The whole hand, fingers or thumbs can be used.

There are different types of pétrissage movement:

- **Picking up** – the tissues are picked up and lifted away from the bone and then released. One or both hands can be used.
- **Kneading** – the muscle is pressed on to the bone using firm movements. This movement can be performed with the palm of one hand or both, or with the pads of the fingers or thumbs.

Uses of pétrissage

- To stimulate sluggish blood circulation
- To aid lymphatic drainage
- To improve condition of skin and hair
- To ease muscular tension.

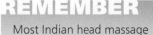

REMEMBER

Most Indian head massage movements will be a type of pétrissage.

Effects of pétrissage

- Blood and lymphatic circulation is increased, encouraging the delivery of fresh oxygen and nutrients to the tissues and an increase in the rate of removal of waste products
- Erythema (redness) is produced
- The elimination of toxins is speeded up
- Sebum secretion in increased, thus moisturising skin and hair.

Tapotement

Tapotement (a French word meaning 'drumming') movements are also known as percussion movements. All tapotement movements are stimulating and so are usually omitted from a relaxing type of massage.
Tapotement movements include:

- **Hacking**, which involves using the side of the hand, known as the ulnar border because of the bone in the forearm called the ulna. The area worked is rapidly struck using alternate hands.
- **Champi**, which is similar to hacking but the hands are placed together as in prayer. With loose wrists, the receiver's back is struck with the little-finger side of the hands.
- **Tabla playing (tapping)**, which is used on the scalp and involves gently tapping on the head with your fingertips, as if playing a piano.

Tapotement movement – champi

Uses of tapotement

- To increase blood circulation to the area
- To warm the area
- To invigorate the receiver
- To tone the muscles.

Effects of tapotement

- Stimulates muscle fibres so muscle tone is improved
- Stimulates sensory nerves on either side of the spine, so it is invigorating
- Increases circulation to the area so that erythema (redness) is produced.

Friction

Two types of massage movement, friction and frictions, although similar in name, are completely different techniques. Friction is the fast rubbing of the skin, which is warming to it. The hands are held stiffly and the palms and fingers are used to rub quickly over the skin.

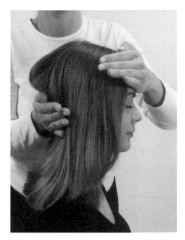

Friction movement

Uses of friction

- To increase blood supply
- To warm an area for further deeper work
- To invigorate the receiver.

Effects of friction

- Brings oxygen and nutrients to the area being worked
- Creates warmth in the area being worked.

Frictions

Frictions involve fairly deep pressure using the finger or thumb. The finger/thumb is pressed on a specific area and there is a gradual increase in pressure. A circular motion with the finger/thumb may also be used. Frictions should cause the skin to rub against structures underlying it, so that one layer of tissue is pressed firmly against another.

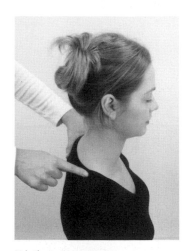

Frictions movement

Uses of frictions

- To relieve tension in muscles, so relaxing them
- To increase circulation and promote healing
- To break down knots in muscles
- To stimulate and invigorate lethargic receivers.

Effects of frictions

- Stimulate the circulation, thereby bringing oxygen and nutrients to the area being worked and producing erythema
- Create warmth in area being worked
- Break down fibrous nodules (knots) in muscles
- Help to invigorate receiver when worked on either side of the spine.

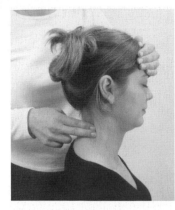

Vibrations movement

TO DO

Research two uses and two effects of the forms of massage movement.

REMEMBER

If a client has come for relaxation, tapotement movements should be limited in use, as these movements are stimulating. More effleurage and stroking movements should be used instead.

Vibration

The hands or fingers of one hand are vibrated so that a fine tremor is produced in the tissues. The tremor is produced by the contraction of the forearm muscles.

Uses of vibration

- Stimulates sluggish lymphatic drainage
- Relieves tension and so induces relaxation.

Effects of vibration

- Promotes relaxation in the muscles worked as it is soothing to nerves
- Relieves pain and fatigue
- Relieves tiredness and lethargy.

Adapting the Indian head massage treatment

Indian head massage can be given to bald clients but certain massage movements involving the hair will obviously need to be left out. Remember not to use too much oil.

Larger clients

These clients may require firmer pressure, but do consult with the client first. You may find that these clients will take a little longer to massage.

Elderly or very slim clients

These clients will probably prefer lighter pressure to be used. Care needs to be taken when massaging over bony areas as it may cause discomfort. Elderly clients can often feel the cold more easily so ensure the room is warm enough. They may need help on to the chair also.

Oils

Indian head massage treatment can be given with or without the use of oils. The main oils used in Indian head massage are sesame, mustard, olive, coconut, almond, sunflower and jojoba. The oils help to moisturise the hair and scalp, which promotes hair growth and slows down hair loss. The treatment can be carried out using vegetable oils mixed with herbs and spices.

REMEMBER

Only qualified aromatherapists should blend essential oils. Unqualified aromatherapists will need to buy preblended oils from shops or wholesalers.

The oils should be unrefined, as the refining process means that the oils are extracted at high temperature, resulting in nutrients being destroyed. The oils should be cold- or warm-pressed and preferably free of additives – look at the product label. With some oils it is advisable to test for allergy, particularly if the client has sensitive skin.

Sesame oil

Sesame seeds are rich in vitamin E and minerals such as iron, calcium and phosphorus, which help nourish and protect the hair and skin.

Uses of sesame oil

- Helps to relieve muscular aches, pains and stiffness
- Moisturises dry skin and hair
- Said to prevent hair from turning grey!

Sesame oil can be used on its own or mixed with other oils such as jojoba and essential oils such as lavender. Sometimes sesame oil may irritate a sensitive skin, so an allergy test may need to be given before using it. Olive oil is an excellent alternative.

HEALTH MATTERS

Allergy testing

Place a couple of dabs of oil behind the client's ear. The oil should be left on for about 24 hours. Often, a reaction will show fairly quickly. It is advisable not to use the oil if there is redness, inflammation or itching.

Mustard oil

Uses of mustard oil

- Relieves tension, pain and stiffness in muscles
- Encourages healthy, glossy hair growth
- Stimulates blood circulation to the scalp so helping to promote warmth; therefore, it is ideal in the winter months.

Mustard oil is often used on its own because its powerful scent does not mix well with other oils. It has been known to irritate skin so an allergy test should be given before using it.

Olive oil

Uses of olive oil

- Helps to moisturise the skin and hair so prevents dryness
- Helps to relieve muscular stiffness and pain.

It is preferable to use virgin or extra virgin oil. Olive oil is a safe oil for the skin and rarely causes irritation; it is therefore an ideal oil to use on children.

Coconut oil

Coconut oil is highly refined, so many of the nutrients are destroyed during the refining process.

Uses of coconut oil

- Softens and moisturises the hair, so is useful for dry, brittle hair
- Encourages healthy hair growth and helps to relieve any inflammation.

Coconut oil can be used on its own or mixed with other carrier oils. It may irritate sensitive skin so an allergy test should be given. It is advisable not to use it on someone with a nut allergy.

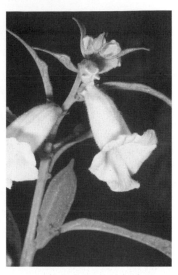

Sesame plant (Sesamum indicum)

REMEMBER

Sesame oil is more easily removed from clothing than most other oils.

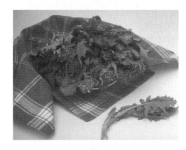

Mustard plant (Brassica juncaea)

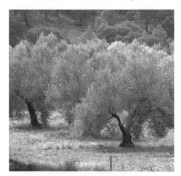

Olive trees (Olea europaea)

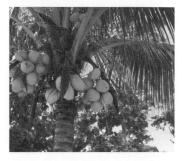

Coconut palm (Cocos nucifera)

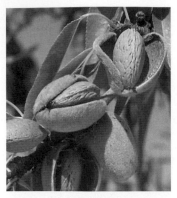

Sweet almond tree (Prunus dulcis)

Sweet almond oil

Uses of sweet almond oil

- Eases muscular tension, pain and stiffness
- Excellent moisturiser for skin and hair
- Promotes healthy, glossy hair as it stimulates the blood circulation to the scalp
- Good to use on clients who have dry hair due to chemical treatments such as colouring or perms.

Sweet almond is a safe oil but it is advisable not to use it on someone suffering from a nut allergy.

Preparation

The therapist

It is important that the therapist presents a professional appearance and manner when carrying out an Indian head massage. Ideally a white tunic should be worn with white or dark trousers; ensure they are clean and ironed. Shoes must be clean and with a low heel. Long hair should be tied back and nails should be cut short. Jewellery should be kept to a minimum. If the therapist gives a bad first impression it is unlikely the client will come back.

It is important to adopt the correct posture when carrying out an Indian head massage. Always keep the back straight and the shoulders relaxed. When carrying out some of the massage movements on the back you may find you need to bend your knees rather than bending at the waist; this will help to prevent strain and injury to your back.

REMEMBER

The whole Indian head massage treatment will take about 45 minutes, including the consultation. Ensure that your client is aware of how long the treatment will take.

The client

Jewellery such as necklaces and earrings should be removed from the client prior to the massage. This will prevent the jewellery accidentally being broken and will help to ensure that the massage flows correctly.

How long will the treatment take?

An Indian head massage treatment will last for about 30 minutes. If a client has a condition such as an aching shoulder, which needs particular attention, you may find that you spend longer on that area than normal. If too much time is spent on one particular area (at the client's request) then you may have to shorten the massage on the face, otherwise you may run over time and be late for the next client.

The massage

Before you start the massage take a minute to get your breathing pattern in line with your client. This will help you maintain concentration and relax the client.

Shoulders

1. Iron down

- Place both flat hands on the shoulders near the base of the client's neck.
- Mould your hands to the shape of the client's shoulders.
- Firmly glide hands along the top of the shoulders and down the upper arms.
- Gently stroke the hands back up the arms and return them to the shoulders near the base of the neck.

(Repeat movement two times.)

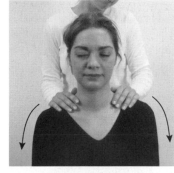

Iron down

2. Friction to shoulders

- Place both hands flat on the client's shoulders.
- Using the fingers of both hands gently rub each shoulder using quick, light side-to-side movements.
- Slide the hands to the upper part of the chest and gently rub using side-to-side movements.
- Slide the hands to the upper part of the back and repeat this movement.

(Repeat movement three times.)

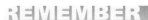

REMEMBER

Friction to shoulders is gentle and soothing; it is good for releasing tension in the shoulders.

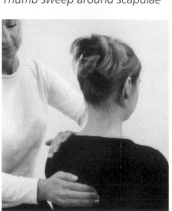

Friction to shoulders

3. Thumb sweep around scapulae

- Place your thumbs at the base of the scapulae (shoulder blades).
- Using both thumbs sweep around the scapulae and across the shoulders (if you prefer you may use one thumb at a time and use the other hand to support the shoulder).
- At the shoulders lift the hands off and return the thumbs to the base of the scapulae.

(Repeat movement four times.)

Thumb sweep around scapulae

4. Finger kneading around scapulae

- Stand to the left of the client.
- Place your left hand on the client's left shoulder (fingers pointing to the back of the client's body).
- Place the pads of the fingers of the right hand at the base of the right scapula.
- Create circular movements in a clockwise direction with the pads of the fingers. Work around the scapula up to the shoulders.
- Stroke your hand back to the base of the scapula and repeat this movement four times.
- Swap sides and repeat movement with right hand on shoulder and use the fingers of the left hand to create circular movements up and around the left scapula. Repeat this movement four times.

Finger kneading around scapulae

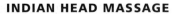

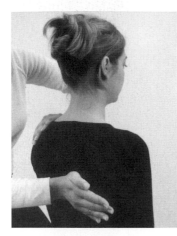

Heel-of-hand knead around scapulae

5. Heel-of-hand knead around scapulae

- Stand to the right side of the client with your right hand on the client's right shoulder, fingers of this hand pointing towards the back.

- Place the heel of the other hand at the base of the client's left scapula.

- Create small circular movements (fairly deep pressure) and work up and around the scapula, working on muscles only, not the bone.

- Lift hand off and return it to the base of the scapula and repeat three times.

- Swap sides and repeat this movement around the client's right scapula with the heel of your right hand.

Can you feel any knots or tension in the muscle being worked? Sometimes you may feel little granules, which indicate tension within the muscle; you will feel them dissolve as you massage.

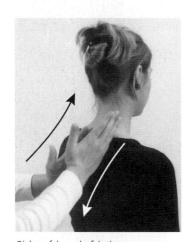

Side-of-hands friction

6. Side-of-hands friction (sawing)

- Place the little-finger sides of both hands anywhere on the upper back.

- Create a sawing action with hands, alternately moving each hand forwards and backwards.

- Work over the whole of the upper back and over the shoulders.

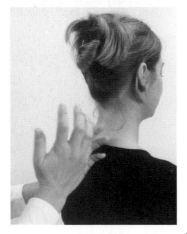

Hacking to upper back

7. Hacking to upper back

- Place the little-finger sides of both hands at the top of the back, anywhere on the trapezius muscles.

- Fingers should not be completely straight but slightly cupped in shape.

- With loose wrists alternately chop with each hand, ensuring pressure is not too great (be gentle over bony areas).

- Work over the whole upper back and shoulder area.

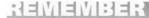

TO DO

Practise this movement on a cushion.

8. Push and pull alternate shoulders

- Place both hands on client's shoulders.
- Slide right hand forwards so it is placed flat on the client's right upper chest region.
- Slide the left hand backwards so it is placed flat on the left side of the upper back.
- Gently push both hands at the same time so that the left shoulder moves forward and the right shoulder moves backwards so a gentle stretch is achieved. Repeat three times.
- Slide the right hand backwards so that it is placed on the client's back and then slide the left hand forward so that it is placed on the upper chest region. Push both hands at the same time and repeat the stretch. Repeat three times.

  Note: This stretch is useful to help loosen tense back muscles.

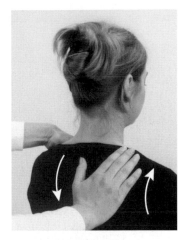

Push and pull alternate shoulders

9. Shoulder pick-up and squeeze

- Place your hands on the client's shoulders, near the base of the neck, fingers pointing forwards and thumb facing the back of the body.
- Push the thumbs towards the fingers. Pick up and squeeze muscles of shoulders between your thumb and fingers and then release.
- Repeat this movement about four times working outwards from the neck and across the shoulders.

  (Repeat whole sequence three times.)

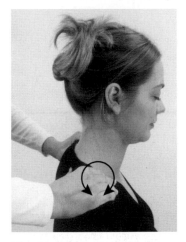

Shoulder pick-up and squeeze

10. Heel push to shoulders

- Cup hands over the client's shoulders, near the base of the neck.
- With the heel of the hands press then release. Use your body weight to create a deeper movement.
- Work from the base of the neck outwards across the shoulders and then stroke hands back again.

  (Repeat the movement three times.)

REMEMBER

If you can feel any knots, use a vibrations massage movement (your forearm muscles are contracted and small tremors are created with the pads of the first two fingers). This will help to disperse the knot).

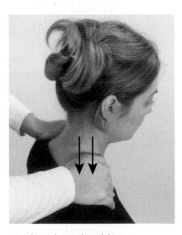

Heel push to shoulders

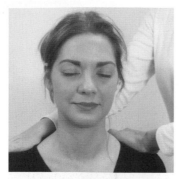

Circular heel-of-hand roll to shoulder

11. Circular heel-of-hand roll to shoulder

- Place both hands on the client's shoulders. The right hand should be near the base of the neck.
- Use the heel of the right hand to create circular movements to the top of the shoulder.
- Begin at the base of the neck and work outwards across the shoulders then back to the base of the neck.
- Repeat the movement with the left hand to the left shoulder.

(Repeat three times on each side.)

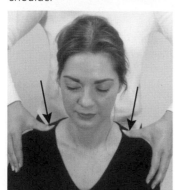

Thumb push to shoulder

12. Thumb push to shoulder

- Place the pads of your thumbs on the outer edge of the client's shoulders.
- Use the pads of your thumbs to push into the shoulder muscles. Release and move about 2 cm towards the base of the neck and again push, then release. Repeat this movement until you reach the neck area.
- Slide the thumbs to the outer edge of the shoulders but place them about 2 cm further back than last time, towards the back of the body. Push and release thumbs again until the neck area is reached.
- Repeat this movement until the whole of the top of the shoulders has been worked over.

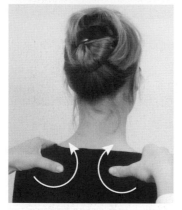

Circular thumb knead to shoulders

13. Circular thumb knead to shoulders

- Place hands on each shoulder, near the base of the neck.
- Use the pads of the thumbs to create slow, circular, clockwise movements.
- Begin at the base of the neck and work outwards across the shoulders. Repeat this movement until the muscles of the upper back and shoulder have been massaged.

Note: Try to work over the whole of the trapezius muscle. Can you feel any knots?

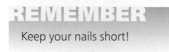

REMEMBER
Keep your nails short!

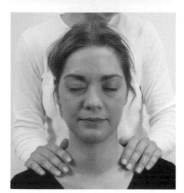

Iron down

14. Iron down

- Place both hands on the client's shoulders, near the base of the neck.
- Firmly slide hands across the top of the shoulders and down the upper arms.
- Lift hands off at client's elbow and repeat the movement.

(Repeat the movement three times.)

Arm massage

15. Pick-up and squeeze to upper arms
- Place each hand at the top of one of the client's arms.
- Squeeze with the hand and then release.
- Slide the hands down the arms, alternately squeezing and releasing.
- When the elbow is reached, stroke back up the arms.

(Repeat the movement two times.)

REMEMBER
Ask the client how the pressure feels – would they like lighter or deeper pressure?

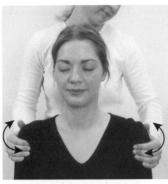

Pick-up and squeeze to upper arms

16. Heel-of-hand circles to upper arms
- Place your hands at the top of the client's arms, fingers pointing forwards.
- Use the heel of the hand to make circular movements.
- Work down the arms and back up again.
- Ensure that the whole of the upper arm (biceps and triceps) is massaged.

(Repeat movement two times.)

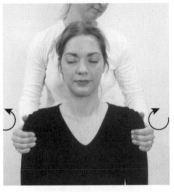

Heel-of-hand circles to upper arms

17. Knuckling to upper arms
- Place your hands at the top of each arm.
- Make a loose fist with each hand, the fingers and knuckles slightly apart.
- Create circular movements with the fist, using the parts of the fingers about 2.5 cm down from the nail to massage and keeping the wrists loose.
- Work over the whole upper arm, particularly concentrating on the biceps and triceps.

REMEMBER
The upper arms can be quite sensitive so do not use too much pressure when massaging.

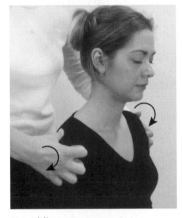

Knuckling to upper arms

18. Forearm roll to tops of shoulders and upper arms
- Place the backs of the forearms on the client's shoulders near the base of the neck. Your palms should be facing upwards.
- Slowly slide the forearms across the shoulders, at the same time rolling the hands inwards so that the palms have turned to face downwards when they reach the tops of the arms.
- Stroke down each of the client's arms with the inside of the forearms.

(Repeat three times.)

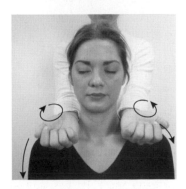

Forearm roll to tops of shoulders and upper arms

Neck

All the neck movements are carried out standing to the side of the client. You may wish to use oil for the neck massage.

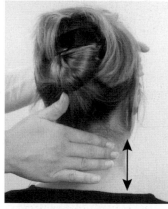

Fingers-and-thumb slide

19. Fingers-and-thumb slide

● Place one hand on the client's forehead to support the head.

● Place the fingers and thumb of the other hand on either side of the vertebrae, on the muscles of the neck.

● Slide the fingers and thumb up the neck to the occipital bone and then slide back down to the base of the neck. You do not need to swap sides for this movement.

(Repeat movement four times.)

20. Three-fingers rub to either side of neck

● Place one hand on the client's forehead to support the head.

● Use the first three fingers of the other hand and place them at the base of the client's neck.

● Gently rub the neck with the fingers creating small up-and-down movements.

● Work up and down one side of the neck and then work on the other side of the neck using the same hand.

(Repeat two times on each side of neck.)

Three-fingers rub to either side of neck

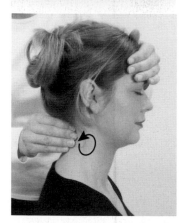

Finger-and-thumb circles to either side of neck

21. Finger-and-thumb circles to either side of neck

● Place one hand on the client's forehead to support the head.

● Place the thumb and fingers of the other hand at either side of the vertebrae at the base of the neck.

● The thumb and fingers slide gently forward to make a small, slow, circular movement and then return to the starting position. Repeat these finger-and-thumb circles and work slowly up to the occipital bone and back down the neck.

(Repeat this movement four times.)

22. Finger-and-heel-of-hand grasp to neck

- Place one hand on the client's forehead to support the head.
- Use the heel of the other hand and fingers to cup and grasp the neck.
- Squeeze and release the muscles at the back of the neck.
- You do not need to swap sides for this movement.

  (Repeat this movement three times.)

Note: If the neck is small, use your fingers and thumb to grasp the neck instead.

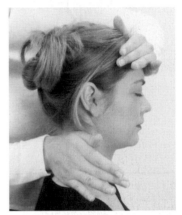

Finger-and-heel-of-hand grasp to neck

23. Heel-of-hand knead to neck

- Place one hand on the client's forehead to support the head.
- Place the heel of the other hand at the base of the neck to the right side of the spine.
- Apply gentle pressure to the neck, creating circular movements with the heel of the hand, and work up and down the right side of the neck for about eight seconds.
- Repeat this movement to the left side of the neck using the same hand.

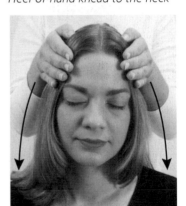

Heel-of-hand knead to the neck

Head massage

24. Effleurage to head

- Stand behind the client.
- Place both hands on top of the client's head.
- Gently stroke hands alternately down the head.
- Repeat until the whole head has been worked.

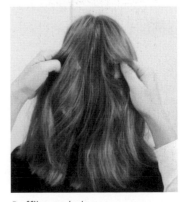

Effleurage to head

25. Ruffling to hair

- Lightly place hands on top of head.
- Open the fingers and draw them through the hair.
- Create wave-like movements, working from the roots to the tips of the hair.

Ruffling to hair

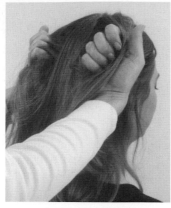

Hair tugging

26. Hair tugging

- Stand behind the client and place your hands on either side of the head.
- Turn hands over with palms facing upwards.
- Comb fingers into the hair.
- Close the fingers together locking the hair in between them.
- Gently tug at the hair and then release.
- Repeat until the whole head has been worked.

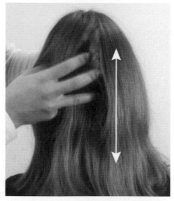

Friction to the head

27. Friction to head

- Stand to the side of the client and support the forehead with one hand.
- Place the heel of the other hand at the base of the head (occipital bone).
- Make small, quick, side-to-side movements using the heel of the hand.
- Work from the base of the head up to the hairline at the forehead.
- Repeat until the whole head has been worked.

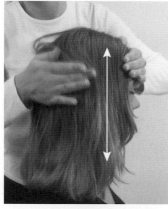

Three-finger rub to the head

28. Three-finger rub to head

- Stand to the side of the client and support the forehead with one hand.
- Place the other hand on the occipital bone.
- Using the first three fingers briskly rub the head, making side-to-side movements.
- Work from the base of the head up to the hairline at the forehead.
- Repeat until the whole head has been worked.

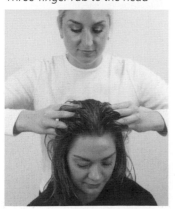

Shampooing to head

29. Shampooing

- Place your hands on either side of the scalp.
- Spread out the fingers and with the pads of the fingers make small, brisk, circular movements as if applying shampoo to the hair and scalp.
- Ensure that the whole scalp is worked.

30. Pétrissage to the scalp

- Place your hands on either side of the scalp.
- Spread out the fingers and with the pads of the fingers glued to the scalp make small, circular movements.
- Lift the fingers away and move to another part of the scalp and work that area, ensuring the whole of the scalp is massaged.
- Complete the head massage by ruffling the hair.

Note: This is an excellent movement for releasing tension in the scalp muscles.

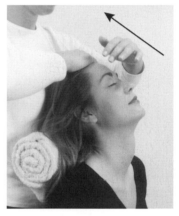
Pétrissage to scalp

Facial

Place a bolster or rolled-up towel behind your client's neck to help support it. You will still be standing behind the client to carry out the facial massage.

31. Effleurage to forehead

- Stand behind the client and use your body to keep the towel in position behind the neck.
- Use alternate palms to stroke slowly up the forehead.
- Work from the right side of the forehead to the left and then to the centre, ensuring that the whole area is worked.

  (Repeat this movement 16 times.)

  Note: This movement is good for relieving headaches and tension.

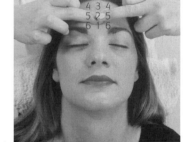
Effleurage to forehead

32. Pressure points to forehead

- Place the middle finger of one hand about 1 cm up from the bridge of the nose.
- Place the middle finger of the other hand on top of that finger to reinforce the movement (no. 1).
- Press and release the fingers and then slide about 1 cm upwards and repeat movement (no. 2).
- Repeat this movement up the forehead until the hairline is reached (no. 3).
- Place middle fingers 2 cm from the top centre of the forehead on either side (no. 4). Press and release fingers.
- Move middle fingers about 1 cm downwards (no. 5). Press and release.
- Slide the fingers down to the final pressure point (no. 6), which is just above each eyebrow.

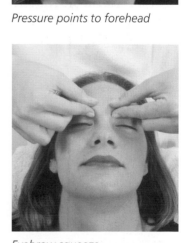
Pressure points to forehead

33. Eyebrow squeeze

- Begin at the part of the eyebrow nearest to the centre of the face.
- Use the first finger and thumb of each hand and gently pinch the tissues of the eyebrow.
- Work slowly across the eyebrows continually squeezing and releasing.

  (Repeat the whole movement three times.)

Eyebrow squeeze

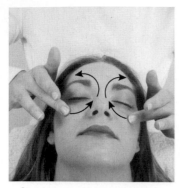

Eye circles with middle finger

34. Eye circles with middle finger

- Place your middle fingers at the outer corners of the client's eyes.
- Gently slide fingers under the eyes and up around the bridge of the nose.
- Bring fingers up and over eyebrows, creating full circles around each eye.

(Repeat three times.)

Note: This is a good movement to help unblock the sinuses.

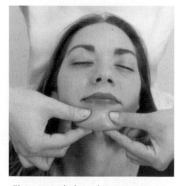

Pressure to cheekbones

35. Pressure to cheekbones

- Place your middle fingers on each side of the client's nose.
- Following the crescent shape of the cheekbones press and release with the middle fingers. Work the top of the cheekbones until you reach the temples. Slide the fingers back to each side of the nose.
- Repeat this movement a little lower down on the cheekbones and then finally work along the lower edge of the cheekbones.

(Repeat whole movement once only.)

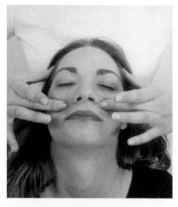

Finger-and-thumb squeeze along jawbone

36. Finger-and-thumb squeeze along jawbone

- Place your thumbs on the client's chin and your index fingers beneath the chin.
- Apply pressure and release.
- Slide fingers about 1 cm outwards and repeat pressures.
- Work from the chin to the top of the jaw bone.

(Repeat this movement three times.)

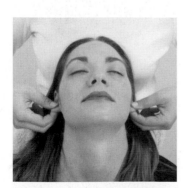

Circular finger kneading to ear

37. Circular finger kneading to ear

- Press your thumbs on the front of the client's ear lobes and the index fingers on the back of the lobes, your right hand working on the client's right ear and the left hand working on the left ear.
- Make small, circular movements with the thumb and finger. As you work up the ears you may have to swap over the finger and thumb and use the finger on the front of the ear and the thumb on the back to massage.
- Work up to the top of the ears and back down again.

(Repeat movement three times.)

38. Circular finger kneading to jaw bone

- Place your fingers on either side of the client's face where the jaw bones meet.
- Use the pads of the first three fingers to make slow, small, circular movements.

(Repeat movement for about 10 seconds.)

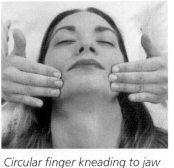

Circular finger kneading to jaw bone

39. Chakra balancing

- Interlock the fingers of your hands. Place the hands about 3 cm from the client's throat – do not place hands directly on the throat.
- Hold the hands in this position for about 10 seconds.
- Move the hands, still interlocked, up to the client's forehead and hold for about 10 seconds.

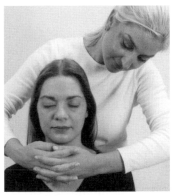
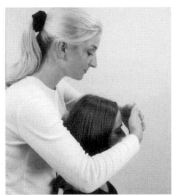
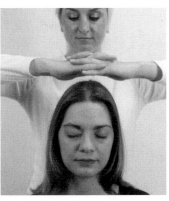

Chakra balancing – throat   *Chakra balancing – forehead*   *Chakra balancing – crown*

- Move the interlocked hands up to the crown of the head, so that the palms are now facing downwards. Hold for about 10 seconds

Note: Even though their eyes are closed many clients report seeing vibrant colours such as purple and orange while the chakras are worked.

40. Prayer effleurage

- Form your hands into a prayer position and then place them on the client's forehead so that the bases of your palms are touching the centre of the client's forehead.
- With the hands still in a prayer position, gently slide hands apart and downwards, so that each hand strokes either side of the forehead. Slide the hands back up again and return them to the prayer position. Repeat this movement three times.
- With hands still in the prayer position, place the base of the palms on the client's chin.
- Slide the hands apart and outwards until they reach the ears. Repeat this movement three times.

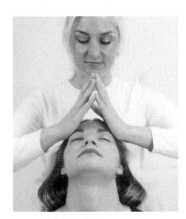

Prayer effleurage

41. Effleurage to head

- Place both hands on the top of the client's head.
- Gently stroke the head with the hands, working downwards to tidy the hair.

(Repeat two times.)

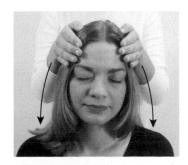

Effleurage to head

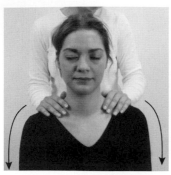

Iron down

42. Iron down

- Place both hands flat on the client's shoulders near the base of the neck.
- Mould your hands to the shape of the client's shoulders.
- Firmly guide hands along the top of the shoulders and down the upper arms.
- Gently stroke the hands back up the arms and return the hands back to the shoulders near the base of the neck.

(Repeat two times.)

Leave your hands on the client's shoulders for a few seconds. Slowly leave the client and observe them and ask them how they feel. Perhaps you could ask if they would like a drink of water. After the client has drunk the water you can give aftercare advice and then book their next appointment.

Aftercare

Aftercare advice should be given directly after the treatment. It is important for the client to follow aftercare advice so that the full benefit of the treatment can be gained.

- The client should be encouraged to rest and relax after the treatment. This ensures that the body is able to heal itself sufficiently.
- The client should drink plenty of water (mineral or tap) or herbal tea to help speed up the removal of toxins from the body.
- Coffee, tea and cola should be avoided as they contain caffeine. Caffeine is a stimulant and therefore will not help the client to relax.
- The client should not smoke or drink alcohol for about 24 hours as the treatment is a detoxifying one and smoking and drinking will reintroduce toxins into the body.
- Heavy meals should be avoided immediately after treatment as blood is diverted to the gut to help with the digestion of the food. The demands of digestion will divert energy away from the healing processes. Light meals such as fruit and vegetables will make an ideal snack.
- It may be wise to ask clients to wait for about 10 minutes after the treatment before driving home, especially if they feel sleepy.

TEST YOUR KNOWLEDGE

1. Why should a heavy meal be avoided immediately after a treatment?
2. In what drinks would you find caffeine? Why should it be avoided after a treatment?
3. What should the client drink after treatment and why?
4. Why should the client not drink alcohol or smoke cigarettes after treatment?
5. What dietary advice would you give a client after treatment?
6. What should a good conditioning treatment for the hair contain?
7. Why do we recommend that a client relax after a treatment has been given?

Chapter 10 Improving your business

Whether you are a salon owner, an employee at a salon or a freelance hairdresser you need to understand how a business makes a profit and keeps customers booking in with you. Advertising, good customer relations and proper use of resources all affect the business's financial success.

This chapter covers the following NVQ level 3 units:
G10 Support customer service improvements
G11 Contribute to the financial effectiveness of the business.

Salon profitability

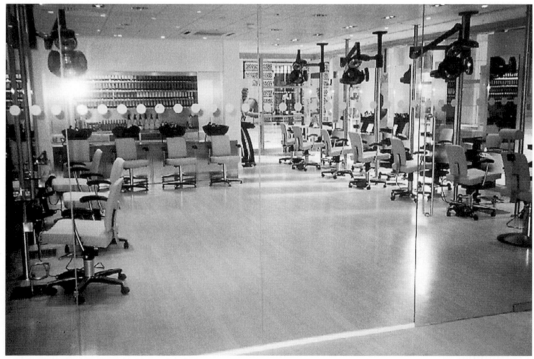

Wella

The financial success of a salon is the responsibility of all staff, from the receptionist and trainee/apprentice to senior management. Contrary to popular belief, salon owners do not use salon takings just to pay staff wages and commission and keep the rest for themselves! The salon takings also go towards the fixed costs of the salon. A salon must have sufficient income to cover salon expenses such as:

- Rent
- Council tax
- Lighting and heating
- Electricity
- VAT
- National Insurance contributions
- Telephone
- Stationery
- Insurances
- Advertising
- Bank charges
- Accountancy
- Sundries, e.g. laundry costs, refreshments
- Cleaning
- Repairs.

TO DO

Using the headings above, try to work out what percentage of salon income would be used by each of the items listed.

The biggest percentage of salon income is taken up by salon wages, rent, council tax and utilities – water and electricity – with other items on the list taking a smaller percentage.

The financial status and prosperity of any salon will be affected by many factors. Seasonal variations will affect client numbers and profits, but the salon overheads will remain the same even when takings are down. This chapter concentrates on ways of ensuring effective use of salon resources and maintaining productivity levels.

TO DO

- *Give examples of resources which may come under each of the categories listed above.*
- *Within your salon structure, to whom would you report any recommendations for improvements in the use of resources?*

Resources

There are many different types of resources used in a salon, including human resources (both staff and clients), stock (for retail and professional use), tools and equipment, utilities, fixtures and fittings, information systems, time, space and, most importantly, money. All of these resources must be used to their fullest potential at all times by all salon staff.

Dealing with resources

When dealing with resources, it is important to remember the following:

- Resources should be used for approved purposes only – for example, the salon telephone should be used for business calls only and not for staff to ring friends.
- Resources must be used to best effect.
- Wastage of products and resources, for example hot water supply, must be minimal.

- The use of resources should comply with organisational and legal requirements. All stock and equipment must be stored, used, handled and disposed of (where applicable) according to manufacturers' instructions, salon and health and safety policies. Staff have legal rights in respect of working hours, breaks and wages.
- The misuse of salon resources could result in wastage, financial loss to the business, damage to tools and equipment, and inconvenience to both clients and staff.

Effective use of resources

To ensure effective use of resources, staff training is essential.

Effective training will ensure that all staff know how and when to use resources correctly, that they comply with health and safety regulations relating to use of resources and can also instruct others in the use of resources – for example, by teaching junior members of staff how to use products and equipment, or by giving clients aftercare advice on products to use in the home.

Stock control

In order for a salon to run smoothly a certain amount of stock has to be carried by the business. The bigger the salon the more stock needs to be kept. Monitoring and rotating the stock is a very important job and one that should be allocated to a particular person in the salon. This avoids wastage and problems arising when stock is short.

Finding information

Information on use of resources can be obtained from various sources:
- Product manufacturers
- Training courses and seminars
- Equipment manufacturers
- Instruction leaflets/manuals
- Salon managers/trainers
- Colleges of further education.

Staff training

Staff training should take place on a regular basis, with health and safety training being updated frequently. Most salons will have staff who have specific responsibilities for training other members of staff, and this training should involve not just teaching new hairdressing skills and techniques, but also how to deal with clients and use new products or equipment.

Legislation relating to resources

There is a large volume of legislation relating to the use of resources in hairdressing, and it is important that all members of salon staff are aware of current laws and that health and safety requirements are enforced at all times (see Chapter 2, pages 40–46). In addition to health and safety legislation, most organisations have their own rules and regulations relating to the use of resources.

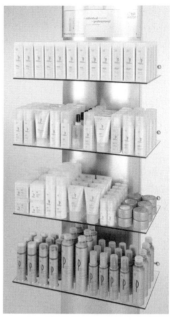

Wella

REMEMBER

CPD or Continual Professional Development is recognised by the Awarding Bodies (City & Guilds, Edexcel, VTCT) as a formal requirement of further staff development and training. Qualified Assessors and Internal Verifiers must keep a log of all practical activities undertaken (a minimum of 30hrs per annum).

REMEMBER

When teaching health and safety procedures or how to use new equipment, keep a written record of the content of each session and who was present.

TO DO

Make up a chart showing who is responsible for the various types of staff training sessions that take place in your salon, under the following headings:
- *Health and safety*
- *Equipment/product knowledge*
- *Practical skills*
- *Client care.*

Staffing structure

Each salon should have a staffing structure, usually consisting of salon owner or manager, senior and junior stylists, trainees or apprentices and, in some cases, a receptionist. Each member of staff should have specific responsibilities within the organisation.

The responsibilities of each member of staff relating to the use of resources should be clearly outlined in their job description. It is also a good idea to display a chart in the staff room showing who is responsible for specific resources. Although the salon owner or manager will usually have overall responsibility, each individual member of staff will need a degree of responsibility in order to carry out their daily salon duties. For example, who is responsible for allocating clients (the most important resource of all) to salon staff? Is this done by the receptionist, or are all staff allowed to take bookings?

TO DO

Make a list of all salon staff and show the responsibilities of each person with regard to salon resources. Remember to address the following questions:
1 Who is responsible for stock control/ordering and dispensing stock?
2 Who is responsible for handling cash/non-cash payments and banking monies?
3 Who is responsible for ensuring tools and equipment are maintained and in good repair?
4 Who is allowed to book appointments?

Problems which may arise

It is important that salons have proper procedures for dealing with any problems that may arise relating to the use of resources, and that all staff are aware of the limits of their authority. They should also know who to refer a problem to if they cannot deal with it themselves.

Listed below are some problems and suggested precautions.

PROBLEMS	PREVENTATIVE MEASURE
Shortage of change in till	Ensure adequate change in float at beginning of day. Keep change in safe in case of emergencies
Client in dispute over payment	Ensure client is informed of salon charges during consultation, before service being carried out
Running out of stock	Ensure stocktaking is carried out on a regular basis – weekly/fortnightly
Discrepancies in amount of takings	Keep accurate records of money taken in till, together with client bill to cross-check
Too much shampoo being used	Ensure staff are aware of correct quantities of shampoo to use
Hot water being wasted at basins	Ensure all staff know to turn water off between shampoos

Productivity in the salon

Poor quality of service, ineffective use of salon resources and failure to make use of opportunities which arise in the salon to offer clients additional services will all result in a **decrease in productivity** within the salon.

Many salons pay staff a commission on their takings and set targets or goals in the form of services to clients or retail sales which the stylist must achieve on a weekly or monthly basis in order to earn their commission.

Setting targets

When setting targets for productivity, it is better to set small goals that can be achieved by staff and gradually increased, than to set unrealistic targets. For example, junior staff could be set retail targets.

Remember to set the targets in negotiation with staff rather than just telling them what you expect – they should be acceptable to both parties. Team goals or targets can be set alongside individual targets, with all salon staff benefiting from their achievement.

Both staff and the salon manager/owner should be responsible for tracking targets throughout the agreed time span, and time should be set aside for regular review meetings. These review meetings are ideal opportunities for individuals to recognise personal strengths and weaknesses within their existing skills and knowledge and enable them to identify any training needs in order to overcome these weaknesses. Ways of identifying one's own strengths and weaknesses include assessing performance against the targets and goals that have been set – are you doing better in some areas than others? Why might this be? Do you need additional training in order to achieve the targets that have been set? If yes, how can you go about getting the training you need? Other ways of helping to focus on strengths and weaknesses include chats and discussions with colleagues and clients. Information on setting targets, identifying strengths and weaknesses and individual and staff training needs is given later in this chapter.

Failure to achieve the agreed targets will affect any commission paid and should be discussed on a one-to-one basis with the individual concerned to find out the reasons for failure. An action plan can then be devised and new targets set.

Repeated failure to achieve targets could result in some form of disciplinary action.

Time and motion study

A good way of analysing the productivity levels of staff in the salon is to carry out a time and motion study.

This involves observing members of staff over a specific period of time, keeping a detailed record of how many times they carry out each type of practical task or service, and how long each service takes.

TO DO

Think of some other problems that could arise relating to resources, and how you could prevent/resolve them.

REMEMBER

If salon targets are not met then:
- Clients may be dissatisfied and the salon image could be damaged
- There may be a loss of revenue for the salon and salaries could be reduced
- In the long term the salon may even close and jobs could be lost

TO DO

Think of some examples of targets that could be set for salon juniors and stylists in your salon.

Week beginning:

	SERVICES				
	Cut and blow dry	Blow dry/set	Perm	Colour	Relaxer
Time allocated:*					
Day/date					
Totals for week:					
Time spent (hours)					

*average time for basic perm/relaxing/colouring techniques – not including processing or drying time
Number of hours worked:

TO DO

Devise some time sheets to give to staff and carry out a time and motion study in your salon.

The time span for this activity should be no less than six weeks and no more than three months. Once all the information has been gathered, you can calculate the average productive time, the percentage of perm, colour and styling work being carried out, the average length of time per service, and the average productive time, per staff member. This will enable you to target quiet times and arrange any special offers and promotions around them.

Increasing productivity

There are many potential opportunities to enhance productivity levels within the salon. These include:

- Staff training
- Promotional events
- Advertising.

Staff training

REMEMBER

Good communication skills are essential. Always be polite, tactful, factual and honest, whether dealing with staff or clients. This will ensure accurate information is given and a professional salon image is promoted at all times.

All staff should undertake regular training in both technical skills and product awareness to enable the salon to offer a complete range of high-quality services. The more technical services and aftercare advice that stylists can offer, the more income they will generate. Training junior staff to carry out simple tasks such as conditioning treatments will also help to increase salon income.

Promotional events

Special offers and promotions should not be restricted to the existing clientele but should be aimed at as wide a cross-section of the public as possible. Try giving existing clients a discount on salon services when they bring a friend to the salon. In order to be successful, promotional activities or events must be organised in advance. Chapter 11 deals with planning and organising promotional events.

Advertising

Using advertisements in local papers and in-house promotional materials will help to promote specific services, staff or products and special offers. When clients respond to a promotional advertisement, this gives the stylist the opportunity to tell them of other services on offer in the salon that might benefit them.

Confidentiality of information

A salon will have many types of information relating to clients and staff, which need to be recorded and updated regularly. The two main ways of recording this information are **manually** through methods such as appointment books, record cards, receipt pads, salon account records, etc., and to use **computerised systems**. Computer packages are available to store client information, staff wage information (pay structures, rates of commission, details of services staff have carried out) and stock control (stock levels and order dates, etc.). Whichever forms of recording and storing information are used by a salon, it is important that all information remains confidential.

TO DO

Find out your salon's rules on confidentiality and what could happen if you break them.

TEST YOUR KNOWLEDGE

1   List the types of resources available in a salon.
2   What could happen if salon resources are misused?
3   How can you ensure correct and effective use of salon resources?
4   Give examples of how productivity levels can be enhanced.
5   What factors could affect productivity levels?
6   What could happen if set targets are not achieved?
7   Why is good communication important?
8   Why should information kept by a salon remain confidential?

The salon team

Who are the team members in a salon? They could be:

- Other trainees
- Junior and senior stylists
- Supervisors
- Managers
- Others working in the salon such as receptionists, beauty therapists, people on work experience, cleaning staff or catering staff
- Voluntary, unpaid helpers such as work placement students from colleges and schools.

REMEMBER

Staff personnel may be full time or part time, permanent or temporary, internal or external and paid or voluntary – they all work for your organisation.

Salons vary in size, so there may be just you and a few other staff in a small salon, or you could be part of a medium-to-large salon of 4–20 people, or even part of a large chain of salons employing hundreds of hairdressers. Wherever you work, you will need to not only do your own work well, but to help and support the rest of the team in an enthusiastic and pleasant manner.

TO DO

Draw up your own line management chart for your salon.

Managing your own workload

Line management
On page 205 is an example of a line management chart which you might like to use as a model when drawing up your own.

Lines of management and each person's limit of authority are important, especially when dealing with client complaints, staff discipline and appraisals.

As a manager or supervisor you need to know:
- Your defined area of responsibility
- How to make decisions and manage budgets within specified limited opportunities, e.g. sending staff on training courses
- How to use resources effectively to achieve specific results, e.g. setting time aside to appraise staff to improve their capabilities and increase business for the salon
- How to allocate work to all staff personnel.

Leadership

Good leaders must have an understanding of how to build a strong team that can work harmoniously and effectively. To do this a leader must have abilities in a number of areas.

Communication

Many clients return to a salon because it has a good atmosphere and the staff are always happy and cheerful. Tension or bad atmospheres in the salon can result in lost clients and poor working relationships.

Continuous improvement

A leader will inspire continuous improvement in the staff by identifying training needs through individual and team appraisals.

Information handling

Staff feedback regarding client services may be obtained in several ways:
- General discussion – informally in the staff restroom during breaks, or formally during staff meetings.
- In a written form, either through staff appraisals (see page 210) or by brainstorming during a staff (or team) meeting. Brainstorming sessions are where everyone offers suggestions which are all written up on a flip chart or noted down, after which they can be analysed and discussed. This information can be itemised and used for future reference.

NAME	POSITION	EXPERIENCE AND QUALIFICATION	LIMITS OF AUTHORITY
Kevin	Owner	20 years hairdressing; A1, A2, V1; Level 2 Hairdressing; C&G Ladies Hairdressing.	Preparing job descriptions. All salon finances. All team problems. Rules and regulations. Health and safety.
Kirsten	Manager	16 years hairdressing; A1, A2; Level 3 Hairdressing; New Zealand hairdressing qualification.	Allocation of staff roles and responsibilities. All technical problems. Interviewing and appointing new staff. Disciplinary procedures. Work allocations. Reports to owner.
Jan	Artistic Director	16 years hairdressing; Master Craftsman; Level 3 Hairdressing; C&G Ladies & Gents' Hairdressing.	Organisation of salon shows, promotions and photographic work. Reports to Manager.
Antonella	Senior Stylist	12 years hairdressing; A1, A2, V1; Level 2 Hairdressing; Level 3 Hairdressing.	Staff trainer. Reports to Manager.
Natasha	Stylist	8 years hairdressing; Level 2 Hairdressing; Level 3 Hairdressing ongoing.	Reports to Manager or Senior Stylist.
Nicola	Receptionist	5 years as receptionist; qualified in secretarial skills.	Responsible for stock control and appointments. Reports to Manager.
Claire	Junior Stylist	3 years, 2 years training; Level 2 Hairdressing.	Reports to Senior Stylist.
Darren	Junior	18 months ongoing; Level 2 hairdressing.	Reports to Senior Stylist.
Andrew	Junior	6 months ongoing; Level 2 hairdressing.	Reports to Senior Stylist.
Jenny	P/T Saturday Junior	6 months ongoing; Level I hairdressing.	Reports to Senior Stylist.

Involvement and motivation

Everyone works for money, which is the strongest motivating force. However, you will have noticed that some people work harder than others! Motivating factors depend on the person's age and where they are in life:

- Mature stylists with their own established clientele may be quite satisfied with just doing their jobs well and see no point in progressing further.
- A young recently qualified stylist may be very ambitious and wish to participate in every training course, promotion, show or photographic session available.

Organisational context

Before you can allocate and supervise another person's work you must find out from your immediate manager exactly what you are allowed to do (i.e. what work is within the limits of your authority). For example, you may feel it would be helpful to carry out a complete salon stock-take, but your manager may have delegated that responsibility to a new manufacturer's company representative.

TO DO

- Before you start to allocate work in the salon, make two lists of all the tasks that need to be done. Make one list for **technical** work such as perms, tints, cuts, etc., and one for **non-technical** work such as reception, salon stock and cleaning duties.
- Once you have made up your lists you need to decide who does what. There are several criteria you must bear in mind:
- **The competence requirements of the work**. For example, a new product from the manufacturer is best trialled on a less busy working day, when staff have time to go through the instructions thoroughly.
- **The competence requirements of the individuals**. For example, it is not a good idea to allocate foil highlighting to a junior until you have seen their work on a model.
- **The existing work commitments of the individuals**. For example, a stylist with a full Saturday clientele would not take kindly to being asked to fit in a wedding party on that day!

Training and development

To support your staff in practical terms you could:

- **Assist salon staff with their technical work** either by offering practical help (e.g. winding their perms or helping with foil highlights) or by providing technical advice (e.g. talking through a colour-correction problem).
- **Participate in staff training sessions** – for example, by either offering to do a demonstration or by planning ahead and rescheduling appointments so that training can take place.
- **Organise a salon promotion** – using your initiative, you could ask your existing manufacturing company to provide an in-house seminar to train staff in the use of new products or equipment.

When helping with the training and development of staff in the salon remember to speak clearly and use language that is easily understood, i.e. not too much jargon. Do not bombard your audience with huge amounts of information all at once; break it down and make sure each point is understood before going on to the next. Repeat your instructions clearly if you need to.

Acting assertively

During conflict situations you need to state your own views and position clearly. A knowledge of both the salon rules and job descriptions helps to clear up any discrepancies.

You will also need to maintain your beliefs, commitment and efforts when there are setbacks and opposition.

Promoting harmony in your team

Generally team harmony is provided by:

- Staff and management accepting and giving feedback in a positive way
- Staff being competent within their job, i.e. not being allocated work that is beyond their skills and capabilities
- Staff supporting each other as part of a team, i.e. not just relying on juniors to help out when necessary, but using their initiative to help each other all the time.

Building teams

As a leader you will need to:

- Make time to help and support everyone
- Give encouragement to stimulate others, and to motivate them, whatever their capabilities
- Evaluate and give everyone feedback to help improve their future performance
- Use your authority and power fairly – don't have favourites!
- Keep everyone informed about whatever progress has been made and what future plans there are
- Invite everyone to contribute to future work developments
- Set achievable and challenging objectives and goals.

Effective communication

You can communicate helpfully with your staff by:

- **Offering your support verbally**, e.g. by helping with technical advice or by praising their efforts
- **Providing practical assistance when necessary**, e.g. by attending to one of their clients if they are behind with their work schedule
- **Listening actively**, by asking questions and rephrasing the person's statements to check mutual understanding, e.g. 'What do you understand by a haircut over the ear?'
- **Identifying what information is needed** by the person you are speaking to, e.g. 'Do you need to refresh your hair colouring knowledge or develop some new advanced techniques?'.

REMEMBER

When dealing with staff problems, always look at the issue, not the person.

REMEMBER

Offer your support, and always provide assistance when necessary. If there is any tidying or cleaning up that needs doing in the salon, if everyone is busy do it yourself. You will encourage team spirit and make other members of the staff more likely to help.

REMEMBER

Always treat others as you would like to be treated yourself.

If you wish to communicate messages to staff, you need to decide:

- **Who needs to receive the message**. If it is everyone, then a staff meeting may be difficult to organise if everyone works different times and on different days. Perhaps a social staff meeting might be more convenient?
- **How to communicate the message**, i.e. verbally or in writing. If the message is verbal, you will need to check that the receiver has understood and will action the message. If the message is written, you will need to make sure that it reaches the right person and is understood by them. Remember also that people communicate all the time by using body language, e.g. someone who avoids eye contact with you may not be accepting the message you are sending.

You must always be sensitive when giving and receiving messages or information to/from your staff, and check that they know what they have to do and how to do it.

Decision making

In the same way that all hairdressers have to project a professional image to their clients and need to give clients their full attention, you, as a supervisor or manager, must never allow salon problems to interfere with your salon management. Remember, the professional image of your salon is at stake. All problems must be dealt with in a calm, considered way.

Use your own experience and look at all the evidence before making a decision.

Personnel issues (i.e. difficulties keeping up with scheduled appointments)

Staff are the salon's major resource, so you must plan carefully and make sure information is passed on to those who need it:

- **Staff holidays**: not only must the clients be rescheduled to suitable members of staff, but you must have a written staff holiday rota so that you know in advance if two or more people are going to be away at the same time.
- **Staff sickness**: always implement a staff sickness procedure, e.g. a statement should be written into job descriptions requiring members of staff who are ill to notify the salon as soon as it opens for business. This will enable you to reschedule all the clients before the start of the working day.

Technical problems (i.e. lack of assistance from team members)

As a supervisor or manager you will often be asked for advice and support. Think back and remember how you felt when you had to wind your first perm and all the perm rods kept falling out and you didn't know which perm lotion to choose! Before giving any advice, take the member of staff to a quiet area away from the client and explain clearly and slowly what you think they should do. Always ask them to repeat it back to you by saying, 'Now exactly which colour and peroxide strength did we decide on?' This will ensure that they have completely understood your instructions and it will reinforce their confidence.

Emergency situations

Health and safety

All salons must have a health and safety policy, including details of evacuation procedures in the event of fire, flood, gas leak, bomb alert or suspicious packages. Careful policy procedures are needed for all of these disruptions to services, and must not only be explained to new staff but regularly confirmed with existing staff.

First-aid procedures

First-aid procedures in the case of major or minor accidents or illnesses must be understood and carried out by all the staff. Most large organisations have a qualified first aider in attendance, and it is a good idea to have a qualified first aider in any salon.

General salon matters

If everyone in your salon has a written job description, laid out in the same way as a line management chart, then it will be clear to them exactly what everyone's job role is. For example, in an emergency whose job is it to evacuate the salon?

Improving customer services

Salon services need to be improved continually, not only for profitability but to inform, motivate, train and develop the staff. Managers and supervisors implement the principles of good practice by identifying needs, planning and contributing to activities and assessing the results.

To motivate staff you need to set them goals, either individually or as a team. However, the goals must be:

- **Specific** – in other words, the goal must be clear. You should not simply say to a junior 'Go and improve'. Improve what? You should say for example, 'You need to improve your perm-winding time.'

- **Achievable** – the goal must be achievable by that person. For example, 'You need to improve your perm-winding time. It took you $2\frac{1}{2}$ hours today; try doing it in two hours next time.'

- **Measurable** – the goal must be measured either by you or the person involved, e.g., 'Look at the clock and note when you started winding that perm, so you can see how long it took you.'

- **Acceptable** – the junior must want to accept the task. For example, before attempting perming again, they might prefer to concentrate on setting and try to achieve a reasonable time for putting rollers in a set.

The staff group could be equally motivated by setting a salon team goal such as increasing the client base by doing a show. The resulting increase in profits would benefit everyone.

Developing the salon (team objectives)

One of the best ways to discover how to improve your services is by asking your clients.

TO DO

If you were absent from the salon through sickness, because you were on holiday or because you were attending a training course, name the person in your salon responsible for:

- *Client complaints*
- *Staff discipline*
- *Rescheduling appointments (due to staff absences)*
- *Obtaining emergency stock*
- *Dealing with technical problems*
- *Salon emergency procedures.*

REMEMBER

Praise is an excellent motivator.

Telling someone off is a negative motivating force.

There are several ways of encouraging client feedback. These include using open-ended questions, having a suggestion box or a client comment box, or using a client questionnaire. An example of a client questionnaire appears on page 211.

If using a questionnaire, remember to hand your client a pen or pencil and something to lean on towards the end of the service when politely asking them to fill it in.

It is important to analyse this information regularly and act upon it to improve your salon services.

Improvements can be made on any scale from adding herbal tea to the salons refreshments offered, adding a new service for clients such as Indian Head Massage or even behind the scenes changes like getting the client records out the day before to save time in the morning or adding a late night to the salons opening hours. Whatever changes are made they should be needed, discussed with the team, training should be given, they should be legal (see chapter 2, page 40) and they should be monitored for their success.

Adding herbal tea to the salons refreshments may not be 'needed' but it is an extra which clients appreciate and would help keep clients loyal. Training should be given to all members of the team on how to make it and present it. Some of the herbal names may be awkward to say so make sure everyone knows how to say them. Then perhaps you could have a client questionnaire to see which the most popular flavours are so you save wasting money on tea that will sit on the shelf.

If you are thinking of adding a new service, apart from the cost of training staff, does the salon have enough room, will the initial outlay of products and advertising be within the salon's budget? Do other salons in the area already offer this service? How will the new service be advertised? And perhaps most importantly will it improve business?

Feedback

Whatever the changes, feedback should be obtained from the clients and staff to measure the success of that change. Clients can be given questionnaires, a comment box or asked open questions. Staff can be asked during their appraisals (see below). Monitoring changes is very important to make sure the change was an improvement and not something which sits on the shelf gathering dust or has caused more confusion or time than before.

Staff development (individual objectives and aspirations)

REMEMBER

All appraisals are **confidential** and provide information only to those who are authorised to have it.

Appraisals

Appraisal systems enable you and the staff to discuss what development is needed for both the salon organisation and for them individually. By setting objectives and goals together you can recommend the best way to achieve them.

A **pre-appraisal** allows for consideration regarding where you are now, an **appraisal** looks at where you are going, and an **appraisal review** enables you to look at whether you have achieved your goals or objectives.

Client Questionnaire

In our salon **you** the client are the most **important person**. We would therefore like to improve our service to you and would appreciate a few moments of your time to complete this simple questionnaire.

Date   _____

Service required   _____

Area where you live   _____

Your age group   15–25 / 26–35 / 36–45 / 46–60 / 61+   *(please circle)*

What time of day did you attend?   9 am–12 pm / 12 pm–2 pm / 2 pm–6 pm / 6 pm–9 pm   *(please circle)*

Was your service …   Excellent/Good/Average/Poor   *(please circle)*

Were you given a free consultation?   Yes/No

Was the salon up to the required standard of cleanliness?   Yes/No

What was the attitude of the staff that attended to you?   Excellent/Good/Average/Poor   *(please circle)*

Did you have to wait for any part of your service?   Yes/No

(If applicable) Was the waiting time acceptable to you?   Yes/No

Are you happy with the quality of service offered at our salon?   Yes/No

Do you consider our salon gives good value for money?   Yes/No

Are you dissatisfied with any part of the service offered?   Yes/No

If yes, briefly describe what was wrong   _____

_____

Would you like any additional hairdressing or beauty services offered in the salon?   Yes/No

If yes, please describe.   _____

If you are a new client, will you return to us?   Yes/No

If no, why not?   _____

If you are a regular client, what is it that keeps you coming to us?   _____

Is there any particular member of staff you find outstanding?   Yes/No

If yes, who is it?   _____

Please place the questionnaire in the box by reception as you leave.

Many thanks.

Pre-Appraisal Questionnaire

Name of Appraisee *Rachel Davies*
Job Title *Senior Stylist*

Current work & responsibilities

Staff trainer
Attends to clients
Long hair specialist

Objectives achieved and outstanding objectives

Achieved   Planning and reviews of model nights for juniors
                   Long hair training sessions

Outstanding objectives – to review and prepare a report on client questionnaires

Which areas of work are you least satisfied with?

My time management

What topics or issues would you like to discuss?

To include hair extensions as a new salon service
To attend a time management course

Development Needs

What skills do you feel need to be developed further?

Feedback and reviews juniors on their training during model nights

What particular training do you require?

Training in the application of both synthetics and real hair extension
Time management training

Name *RACHEL DAVIES*   **Signature** *R Davies*   Date *3/11/03*

Appraisal Questionnaire

Name of Appraisee   *Rachel Davies*   Job Title   *Senior Stylist*

Name of Appraiser   *Stephanie Henderson*   Line Manager   *Noel Otley*

Date appointed to present post   *September 2001*

Appraisal Cycle From   *November 2003*   to   *November 2004*

Current work & responsibilities

Staff Trainer

Attends to clients

Long hair specialist

Which areas of work are you least satisfied with?

Time Management

Negative feedback from some juniors when criticised during training

What objectives or goals have been achieved in the last appraisal cycle?

Fully booked client column 3 weeks in advance

Planned and reviewed model nights for juniors

Presented 3 long hair training sessions for staff

What objectives or goals are still to be achieved?

To review and prepare a report on the client questionnaire

To include hair extensions as a salon service

To improve my time management

To improve feedback during training the junior staff

What action needs to be done to achieve them?

To collate all questionnaires and extract the strengths and weaknesses

To attend training in hair extensions for both synthetic and real hair

To attend a time management course

To attain D32 D33 TDLB training certificate

What other achievements have been made?

Attended a first aid course and achieved Life Savers Certificate – St Johns Ambulance Brigade

Attended three manufacturers courses to update colour, perm and cutting skills

Objectives/Goals to be achieved within this appraisal cycle

Objectives/Goals	Action	Criteria for Success	Time Scale
To prepare a report from the client questionnaire	To collate all questionnaires and extract the strengths and weaknesses	Complete report based on questionnaires	End of Jan 2004
To offer hair extensions as a salon service	To attend a hair extension course and become competent	Hair extension Diploma	End of March 2004
To improve my time management	To attend a time management training course	Decrease in client waiting time reviewed through client questionnaires	End of June 2004
To attain A1 and A2 Assessors Training Certificate	To register with a local college and City & Guilds, attend training courses and complete the work	A1 and A2 Certificates	End of October 2004

Personal Development Plan

What are your career objectives?

> To become a salon manager within the next three years
> To increase my client takings by 20%

What additional training/knowledge/skills are needed by the appraisee?

> Guidance with preparing client questionnaire report
> To practice in the use of hair extensions on a tuition head
> To be able to transfer time management knowledge to a client column
> To understand the amount of work required to obtain the A1 and A2 Certificate

What actions need to be taken to meet these training needs?

> To discuss client questionnaire with line manager
> To research the cost of hair extensions for practice
> To prepare a list of questions regarding client columns to take to the time management course
> To discuss with my local college tutor the course requirements of obtaining both A1 and A2

Comment by Appraiser	Comment by Appraiser's Line Manager
Excellent achievements, well done	Well done, we will try to help fund most of your new training needs
Signature S Henderson Date 10/11/03	Signature N Otley Date 18/11/03

Comment by Appraisee	Signature of Appraiser and date when returned
Thanks for being so helpful, I can't wait to start	25/11/03 S Henderson
	Signature of Appraisee and date when returned
Signature R Davies Date 12/11/03	26/11/03 R Davies

Identifying staff needs

A pre-appraisal questionnaire given to staff a few weeks before an appraisal will identify staff development needs and can be presented at an appropriate time during appraisals.

During the completion of the pre-appraisal questionnaire staff will have an opportunity to contribute to their own development needs – for example, they will be able to reflect on both past and future training. A full appraisal needs time – usually $1\frac{1}{2}$–2 hours in a quiet area, with no interruptions, and gives both the appraisee and the appraiser time to consider what development needs are relevant and realistic, and to take account of team and organisational constraints (such as salon policies, time and money).

The individual development needs can then be considered against the needs of the other staff. You may then decide, perhaps, that a specialist giving 'in-house' training to all staff will be more cost-effective than individual training courses.

Integrating individual and team objectives

As a manager or supervisor you may need to prioritise the identified team and individual needs because of financial and time constraints.

Team and organisational **values** may be different from the **training needs**; for example, an organisational value may be that the salon always closes on Sunday, but the training need may be that a full day's staff training can only be delivered on a Sunday.

Once all the team and individual needs have been identified you may need to gain agreement from:

● Team members

● Other managers or colleagues working at the same level

● Line managers (above your level)

● Specialists (such as manufacturers' trainers).

You will need to use your prioritised list of training and list the strengths and weaknesses of each. For example:

Individual training needs
Strengths:

● Implementing model nights for junior staff

● Implementing long-hair training sessions for all staff

● Managing a full client column.

Weaknesses:

● Unable to offer hair extension services to clients

● Coping with negative feedback from some junior staff in training

● Running late with appointment system.

TO DO

Look at the example of a completed pre-appraisal form, then list which developments apply to team objectives and which apply to individual aspirations. Make a list of each one then compare it with the individual job descriptions and the team development needs.

TO DO

List three different organisational values against three different training needs.

Team training needs
Strengths:
- Well-motivated and enthusiastic team members
- All staff trained to a minimum of NVQ L2 standards
- Ongoing training by a specific manufacturer in current products.

Weaknesses:
- No staff able to offer hair extension services
- Client waiting time increased due to poor time management
- Assessment feedback techniques causing ill feeling amongst some trainees.

Integrating appraisals into development planning needs

A good development plan needs to utilise appraisals, and the following are examples of training that could take place:
- Hair extension training for one member of staff to cascade to others (to a specialist such as a manufacturer's trainer and to team members)
- Time management training for key members of staff (to a line manager)
- A1 and A2 training for the staff trainer (to colleagues working at the same level).

Organisational constraints
The salon's developmental planning needs may be at odds with the organisational constraints for example:
- **Time** – salons are busiest at holiday times and staff training may be better carried out at quiet periods
- **Finance** – the salon's training budget could be enhanced by sponsorship from a manufacturer
- **Line management** – senior staff may be intimidated by junior staff offering specialist training, therefore a senior member may need the initial training to cascade to others.

Implementing development plans

To ensure equal access by enabling every member of your team to be involved, development plans must take account of:
- **Team members' work activities** – e.g. a training evening after a busy day when staff are tired is not as beneficial as using a period when the salon is quiet
- **Team members' learning abilities** – e.g. it is not beneficial to give advanced training to junior staff who have not completed their initial training
- **Team members' personal circumstances** – e.g. staff who have a long distance to travel to work may not be able to attend an early morning training session.

The manager's contributions

There are three ways in which you could contribute personally towards planning developments.
- By taking part in the development activity yourself through issuing briefing documents e.g.

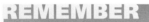
REMEMBER

All development plans must be agreed with everyone involved to create harmony and a positive communication system.

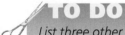
TO DO

List three other reasons why you should consider the above points.

```
                          Memo
To      All Staff
From    Stephanie Henderson - contact  extension  223 re any
        queries
Date    27/11/03
Re      Staff training session on long hair
        Wednesday evening 06/01/04 6.30pm — 8.30pm
All staff are required to bring one model at 6.30pm with hair
below shoulder length which has been washed the day previously.
The salon will supply pins, grips and ornamentation. We will
continue to practise for our bridal theme.
Looking forward to seeing you there.
Signed
                   S Henderson
             Stephanie Henderson
```

● By providing opportunities for learning at work, for example:

```
                          Memo
To      All Staff
From    Stephanie Henderson - contact extension 223 re any
        queries
Date    28/11/03
Re      Staff training on long hair
The salon's appointment book is becoming too busy to hold this
session on the date arranged yesterday — and this has been
confirmed by memos from several staff members. I have therefore
rescheduled the training day for 8th January. Please make a
note of this in your diaries.

Signed             S Henderson
             Stephanie Henderson
```

● By modifying development activities to take account of the feedback you have
received, for example:

Notice to all Staff

Client Questionnaire

Please ensure that each of your clients is given the opportunity to complete
the enclosed sample of the client questionnaire form during the forthcoming
week. Please place the completed forms in the box by reception.

We shall analyse the results and decide if we need to provide any further
staff training in customer service.

Please call me on extension 223 if you have any problems or queries.

From Stephanie Henderson

Manager

Choosing the development activity

Different development activities, such as offering hair extensions as a salon service, improving time management, obtaining their Assessor's qualifications, need different considerations before any decisions to go ahead can be made.

- The team members:
  - Is the activity suitable for their clientele?
  - Would they need considerable practice?
- The type of development activity:
  - Is it cost effective?
  - Is it time effective?
- The manager's own abilities:
  - Is training needed beforehand in organisational or motivational skills?
- The situation:
  - Is there enough space in the salon for the training?
  - Will there be enough suitable models for the training?

Once all of these factors have been considered:

- provision of information, e.g. from the appraisals and client questionnaires
- instructions, e.g. from a health and safety policy document
- skills and training, e.g. hair extensions
- provision of learning opportunities at work, e.g. training in long hair

and discussed with all staff personnel, then time must be allowed for feedback (evident in the memos or notices to staff) before implementation.

Presenting ideas for planning developments

The ideas that have been gathered from individual appraisals, results of client surveys, informal and formal staff meetings and published literature about available training courses must be collated and prioritised for formal presentations.

Initially agreement should be gained from the authorised people, i.e. the training personnel involved, then the higher-level line manager. Colleagues at the same level should then be informed and, finally, the rest of the team.

When agreement has been gained from all those involved then the development plan can be implemented.

The assessment of development objectives

Reviews are important in the development planning process because, by looking at the success criteria of the stated goals and objectives, they will enable the manager to focus on whether knowledge and skills and performance at work have improved.

Improvement may be measured by:

- **Testing knowledge or skills** through identifying agreed criteria, e.g. attaining A1 and A2 assessors' awards
- **Observation of performance at work**, e.g. analysing the client's questionnaires regarding waiting times

- **Appraisal discussions**, by completing an appraisal review document.

Staff can contribute to their own progress by taking part in an appraisal review, making any comments and signing to say that the review is valid.

Salon personnel must be confident that all assessments are confidential and that documents are available only to authorised people. This would help to create harmony in the team.

All assessment results should be discussed with the individuals or teams being assessed, then the higher-level line manager, then (if appropriate) colleagues working at the same level as the manager, and finally with any specialists involved.

Remedial actions

Hopefully, by using the effective communication techniques described in this chapter, you will have given constructive feedback and have a happy, motivated work team. However, problems can occur. For instance:

1 You have allocated someone a training job and they have not carried it out at all

There are two possible solutions to this:

- You must reallocate the training work to someone of equal competence.
- You need to counsel the person and explain how important it was that the job was done, and then refer the matter to your immediate manager. This must be done privately – never in front of other staff.

2 You have allocated someone a training job and they have not carried it out in the way you specified

The usual reason for this is that you did not explain the job clearly enough. The answer is therefore to provide more support by explaining it again, giving the person some instructions to read, or by asking someone else to demonstrate the skill to them again.

REMEMBER

All of the purposes that an assessment may have must **be agreed** with the salon personnel and specialists (if involved). For example, the results of a client questionnaire survey which suggest that staff training is needed in customer service requirements must be agreed before training is commenced.

REMEMBER

All assessments must be valid, authentic, current, reliable and sufficient and must be assessed against agreed goals.

TEST YOUR KNOWLEDGE

1 Why is it important to encourage salon personnel to develop effective salon improvements?

2 How can the manager or supervisor contribute towards these improvements?

3 Why should you provide salon personnel with opportunities to contribute to identifying their own development needs?

4 Describe the differences between development needs which may meet team objectives and those which meet individual aspirations.

5 How can the manager or supervisor prioritise between team development needs and individual aspirational development needs?

6 Describe the implications of comparing team development values with team development training needs.

7 How could you present development needs in a positive way to the following:
- Team members
- Colleagues working at the same level
- Line managers
- Specialists

8   What are the principles of good practice in planning the development of teams and individuals?

9   Describe how an appraisal system can be integrated into the salon's developmental planning needs.

10 List two organisational constraints that may influence the salon's developmental planning needs and describe how they could be incorporated into the planning process.

11 Why and how do development plans have to be agreed with everyone involved?

12 Why should developmental plans take account of:
    - Team members' work activities
    - Team members' learning abilities
    - Team members' personal circumstances

    and how could you take these into account?

13 List three different contributions that the manager can make to the various activities for team members.

14 How could the manager decide on what contributions to make towards developmental activities relating to:
    - The team members
    - The type of developmental activity
    - The manager's own abilities
    - The situation?

15 How could the manager ensure that their own contribution is meeting the agreed objectives and plans?

16 How and why should the manager monitor and review development activities and note the feedback of those taking part?

17 What are the correct procedures for presenting ideas and contributions to planning developments?

18 Why is it important to assess team members' development?

19 Why should the range of purposes of an assessment be agreed with all salon personnel and specialists?

20 State the reasons why team members should contribute towards the assessment of their own progress, giving examples of how this could be done.

21 Describe the principle of objective and fair assessment.

22 Detail how you could implement the following assessment methods objectively and fairly:
    - Testing of knowledge and skills
    - Observation of performance at work
    - Appraisal discussions.

23 Why is confidentiality important during assessment procedures?

24 Describe the procedures for reporting assessment results.

Appraisal Review

Name of Appraisee   *Rachel Davies*

Job Title   *Senior Stylist*

Date of Review   *June 2004*

Review of Objectives Set

Objectives which have been achieved should be listed. Where objectives have been changed new ones should be agreed. All objectives should be achievable and measurable.

Objectives/Goals	Action	Criteria for Success	Time Scale
To prepare a report from the client questionnaire	To collate all questionnaires and extract the strengths and weaknesses	Complete report based on questionnaires	End of Jan 2004
To offer hair extensions as a salon service	To attend a hair extension course and become competent	Hair extension Diploma	End of March 2004
To improve my time management	To attend a time management training course	Decrease in client waiting time reviewed through client questionnaires	End of June 2004
To attain both the A1 and A2 Assessors Certificate	To register with a local college and City & Guilds, attend on training courses and complete the work	A1 and A2 Certificates	End of October 2004

Review of Training Development Needs

Training development carried out by appraisee since last review

> *Direction regarding preparing client questionnaire summary results from line manager*
> *Attended hair extension course in February 2004*
> *Enrolled and attended local college to attain A1 and A2 certification*

Training and development requirements which have been changed since last review

> *Time management issue now being resolved through closer supervision of client appointment schedules*

Action which will be taken to meet changed requirements

> *Discussion forum with all staff personnel to analyse client timings for the appointment schedules*

Criteria used to assess whether training and development which takes place is a success

Client surveys indicated that some staff need to obtain customer service NVQ
Hair extension services utilised by clients
Three summative assessments obtained towards A1 and A2 certification

Comments by Appraiser

You have worked very hard in all areas and are achieving your planned goals.

Signature *S Henderson*   Date   *12/6/04*

Comments by Appraisee

I am pleased with my attainments to date and hope to complete my A1 and A2 by September 2004

Signature *R Davies*   Date   *12/6/04*

Comments by Appraiser's Line Manager

Very good achievements, you have also helped the team development by highlighting both reception and customer care development needs. Well done.

Signature *N Otley*   Date   *26/6/04*

Chapter 11 Promotions and shows

Fantastic opportunities are available to any hairdresser who wishes to display their hairdressing skills either in front of a live audience or in front of the camera lens. Special organisational skills, fast thinking, creativity and the ability to keep a cool head when everything falls apart are attributes needed for large promotional activities. Of course not all promotions are 'lights, camera, action!' A promotion can be a display in the window of the salon or a stand at a local wedding fair. Either way this chapter will help you learn the skills needed for a good promotion.

This chapter covers the following NVQ level 3 units:
H24 Develop and enhance your creative hairdressing skills
H32 Contribute to the planning and implementation of promotional activities.

Creative thoughts

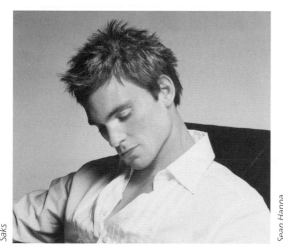

Saks

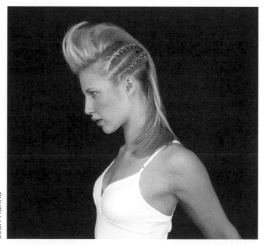

Sean Hanna

Creative thoughts do not have to be completely original. They can be based on developing existing styles and ideas to create something slightly different. Many factors can spark creativity, including images from television and films, historical or artistic images, pictures of film and pop stars, or from the environment or nature.

Altering and modifying classic and fashion styles, adapting an avant-garde/alternative concept through creative use of colouring, perming and cutting techniques – these are just some ways in which hairdressers use artistic expression in their work.

TO DO

Put together a scrapbook of what you consider to be creative images, using pictures taken from magazines, fashion and history books, etc.

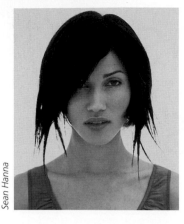

REMEMBER

When creating an image, you need to relate it to the basic principles of:
- Design – which requires an understanding of symmetry and asymmetry
- Scale – which requires an understanding of relative size
- Proportion – which requires an understanding of the weight, balance and distribution of the media used.

Creating images

There are many opportunities to be more creative with your work. They include hair and fashion shows, photographic sessions, special occasions such as weddings, or hairdressing competitions.

Hair and fashion shows
Hair shows provide many possibilities for creating artistic and creative images but require very detailed planing and preparation in order to be successful.

Special occasions
A classic example of a special occasion is a wedding. Creating a hairstyle for a bride often involves working with long hair and hair accessories. There is often scope to transform the client to create a total look which complements the wedding ensemble.

Hairdressing competitions
There are many categories of hairdressing competition, including commercial, avant-garde and fantasy styling. They give the hairdresser the opportunity to be highly creative, making use of strong colours and added hairpieces and creating a total look for the model, including clothing, accessories and facial or body make-up.

Photographic sessions

Producing a portfolio of your own work is a good way of promoting your hairdressing skills and creative talents to both existing and potential clients and employers. Photographs can also be submitted to hairdressing magazines for publication, which can help promote public recognition of your work.

Points to consider when planning a photo shoot

When planning a photo shoot remember to take the following into consideration:
- Budget constraints
- Photographer
- Models
- Location
- Backdrops
- Lighting

Budget constraints
These will influence the scale of your photo shoot. Does your budget allow you to hire a photographer, or will you be taking your own shots? Can you afford to pay for professional models or will you have to use clients or friends? Remember to set aside some of the budget for clothes, accessories, hairpieces, etc.

If you decide to use a professional photographer, choose someone who has experience of fashion and beauty photography. Looking through **Yellow Pages**, checking out **photo credits in trade journals and magazines** and contacting salons that produce their own photography are some ways of finding a photographer.

When interviewing photographers, always ask to see their **portfolios** and question them about work they have done for other salons/stylists.

Find out what the fees will be and whether they include **film and processing costs**, as these can often be additional. Some photographers have **assistants** who may be willing to do the work free, or at a reduced rate, in order to gain experience.

Models

If your budget allows, contact model agencies and explain the type of models you are looking for. Some model agencies can be reluctant to supply models if you wish to totally change their hair by cutting or colouring as this could affect any further modelling jobs. Models who are relatively new may be willing to pose free in return for shots to include in their own portfolios.

Whether you use professional models or find your own, always use more than one model during a session. You cannot predict how things will turn out and restricting yourself to one model could mean the shoot may not produce any good results. If using clients, friends or colleagues as models, remember the following:

- What someone looks like in 'real life' is no guide to how they will look on film. Some people can be extremely attractive yet photograph poorly. A good tip is to take a Polaroid photo before the actual session and assess the results.
- If you have someone with quite hard but interesting features, try photographing them in black and white, which can soften the features.
- When choosing models, remember that the camera can make people appear heavier and larger than they are, so take time to choose models who are well proportioned.

Location

If you use a professional photographer, ask if they have a studio. If you prefer to work from your salon, check that this is alright with them. If you choose to take shots outdoors, remember that elaborate backgrounds and scenery can detract from the subject of your photographs.

If you use a location or have to go to the photographer's studio, remember to take all the equipment and accessories you will need with you. It is a good idea to make a list in advance.

Backdrops
When planning your photographs, think about where and how they will be used. Do you want to take head shots only or full frame? There are many types of backdrops that can be used: seamless paper and fabrics which will drape well are just two examples. Discuss colours and textures with your photographer.

Lighting
A professional photographer should be able to advise you on the most suitable lighting. This will vary depending on what you are showing – hair colour, shape, or texture. Do you prefer natural or artificial light? Are you taking colour, black-and-white shots, or both?

REMEMBER

The roles of colleagues involved in the photo session should be clearly defined and accurately communicated. See Chapter 1 on communication skills.

Developing your ideas

Once you have identified your opportunities for creating images, you must come up with, and develop, some specific ideas.

Ideas can come from many sources – hair and fashion magazines, brainstorming sessions with colleagues based around themes such as history, the 1970s, etc. Often the source will depend on the event or occasion, or the setting in which you want your work to be seen.

Once the ideas have been decided upon, they can be developed further. Remember that one idea can often spawn several others, and it is important to keep comprehensive, accurate and up-to-date records showing the planning, design and presentation of your ideas for future reference.

It is a good idea to compile a **portfolio** and include in it any plans, sketches, diagrams, illustrations and magazine cuttings. You can also include budget information, results of discussions and consultations with those involved, resources needed, such as equipment, materials (added hair, accessories, clothes, make-up) and additional media requirements. It is also important to include information on where resources can be obtained – names and telephone numbers of suppliers and contacts, whether items have to be purchased or can be borrowed, perhaps those working on the idea with you have materials or equipment that could be used. Remember to record it all.

Make your own mood boards to show colours, themes and ideas by cutting pictures from magazines. This will keep you focused on your original ideas.

Adapting ideas
Remember that you can alter or modify your original ideas as required, depending on the opportunities selected.

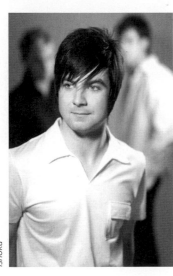

Ishoka

- Try to create styles that can easily be transformed by adding hairpieces or accessories. This will save time and allow many different looks to be created without much effort.
- Try duplicating the same style on different models – this can often produce effective results.

Making your own hairpieces using real or synthetic hair is a cost-effective alternative to buying pre-prepared hairpieces. Hanks of real and synthetic hair can be purchased quite reasonably from wholesalers or by mail order, and both types of hair come in a variety of shades and tones which can be colour-matched to a model's natural hair.

Hair extensions can also be added to a model's hair to provide length and bulk, thus allowing a wider range of creative images to be produced (colour plate 7).

Trade magazines and exhibitions such as Salon International frequently promote suppliers of hair extension systems that use either synthetic or real hair.

Evaluating ideas
The suitability of the ideas chosen and their progression can be evaluated through discussion and consultation with colleagues. Look at what you have created and analyse its suitability. Are there any changes you need to make? Remember to

encourage constructive comments and be willing to take on board what others involved in the project have to say.

Large-scale projects

When undertaking any large-scale projects it is important to consider:

- **Benefits to the salon**. These could include a higher profile within the industry and with the general public. This in turn could help to attract new staff, which might increase salon business and lead to further opportunities. See Chapter 10.
- **Benefits to you**. These could include wider recognition of your own skills, an increase in your client base, a higher profile in the salon, further job and career development and possible increase in salary.

TEST YOUR KNOWLEDGE

1   Give examples of different forms of artistic expression.
2   Where could you find inspiration for creating artistic images?
3   Give examples of ways of coming up with creative ideas.
4   How could you record your ideas and their development?
5   List the benefits to yourself and your salon of promoting artistic images.
6   Where could you find information on false hair/hair extensions?
7   List the things you need to consider when planning a photo shoot.
8   Give examples of forms of evaluation that can be used.
9   Why is it important to set and work to a budget?

Setting objectives

In order to increase salon business, it is essential to take an active part in promoting the salon, the staff and the services you offer.

When arranging any type of promotional activity it is important to set out and plan the objectives or outcomes of the activity. The objectives are to:

- Plan the work for your team or individual staff members
- Assess the work for your team or individual staff members
- Give feedback on the work to all your team members.

Why do a promotion?

The main reasons for promoting a salon are:

- To promote and enhance the salon image
- To make clients aware of the services the salon offers
- To attract new clients
- To encourage existing clients to return
- To motivate staff for personal growth and achievement and to become part of a successful team.

Discussions with management and colleagues will help identify areas that need development and establish the objectives of your promotional activity.

How can you promote your salon?

There are many ways in which to promote a salon.

Short term
- Displays, e.g. retail display in salon
- Special offers, such as:
  - free product samples
  - discount prices on services.

Medium term
- Advertising, for example:
  - local newspapers
  - local television/radio
  - leaflet drops
  - within salon, using promotional posters/photographs of work by staff
- Demonstrations, e.g. to professional and non-professional groups
- Shows, e.g. to small and large groups (school fashion shows, Women's Institute, Girl Guides).

Objectives
Once you have decided to promote your salon it is important to have a set of objectives. This can be referred back to when everyone starts to go off on a tangent and gets carried away with the planning, as creative people tend to do. A good way to write objectives is the SMART way:

TO DO

List the ways in which you could best promote your salon, and the main objectives of each method.

- **Specific** – statements must be specific, clear and plain. Everyone needs to understand the plan.
- **Measurable** – targets and goals must be defined such as finish time, size, budget, audience.
- **Achievable** – goals and targets must be achievable, but also not too easy.
- **Realistic** – objectives must be real – not ideal. Work within the constraints of budget, venue, expertise, resources.
- **Time-bound** – you must have a start time/date and finish time/date and stick to it.

Targeting the promotion
The nature of the target group you wish to attract will influence the promotional activity you choose to present.

When planning a promotional activity, consider the following questions:
- Do you want to attract the general public in order to expand your client base? If so, what age groups do you want to appeal to – a specific age range, or a wider cross-section of the community?
- Do you want to attract female clients, male clients, or both?
- Will your promotion be aimed at new clients, existing clients or both?
- What is your product/service? Do you have a clear idea of what, or who, you are trying to promote?

- When will the promotion take place? Will clients need advance notification, e.g. for a show demonstration?
- Why should they buy/use the product or service? What are the benefits to them? (Remember that listing the benefits of the product is an important part of selling.)
- How is it to be used? In the case of a product or service, clients and customers need information.

Important points to remember

To ensure the success of any promotional activity, planning and preparation are vital to gain everyone's support and commitment. It is a good idea to have a detailed plan showing what is to be done, by whom and when. It should include:

- Dates and times of any team meetings
- Jobs to be carried out, and by whom
- Responsibilities of those involved, that is:
  - those with line responsibility – who have to plan and report back to their line manager
  - those with functional responsibility – who have specific functions within various areas of work and may not be part of the line management, e.g. a part-time specialist media consultant
- Rehearsal dates (if required)
- Deadline dates.

It could also include information on available resources and budget details. Remember to update your plan on a regular basis, making a note of any changes.

Motivating staff

Involving members of staff in putting together and presenting any form of promotional activity is a good way to motivate them.

The following are proven motivators:
- Being given responsibility with an element of independence
- Being given work that is creative and challenging
- Having scope for personal growth and achievement
- Being part of a successful team.

If staff are motivated, they are more likely to work hard, and if they are given specific roles to carry out during the promotional activity, this will help ensure its success and give those involved a sense of achievement.

Resources

The next step is to consider the resources you will need in order to carry out your promotion successfully. These usually fall into three categories:
- Staffing
- Tools and equipment
- Promotional materials and products.

Uxbridge College Hair and Beauty Show

Venue	Hayes site
Date	Sunday 25 April 2004
Time	Doors open 7.00 pm
Seating capacity	200/250

Student responsibilities

Beauty therapy students	Make-up
FT 1st Year Hairdressers	Assisting
FT 2nd Year Hairdressers	Preparation of models
P/T Level III Hairdressers	Organising models/clothes/accessories/preparing models

Staff responsibilities

Line responsibility

Claire Jones	Co-ordinating Beauty Therapy students
Kirsten Harjette	Co-ordinating 2nd Year students, liaising with Marketing, Lighting and Sound

Co-ordination functional responsibility

Stephanie Henderson	Liaising with sponsors and photographers

Show structure

Four main sections:

7.30 pm	Start: 20-minute Introduction
	Scene 1: Black-Sleek lines
	Scene 2: White
Break for refreshments	*30 minutes*
8.20 pm	Level III: Historical/High Fashion and Fantasy
8.35 pm	Scene 3: Black and White
	Scene 4: Colour and Finale

TO DO

- *Using your chosen promotional activity, list the various jobs that need doing.*
- *Match your staff/colleagues to each role.*

Staffing

When delegating tasks, always consider the strengths of the individual(s). Remember that you are also giving each individual authority and it is important that everyone involved is aware of the limits of their authority, what their responsibilities are and when they will be needed.

Tools and equipment

The tools and equipment required will be dependent on the type of promotional activity you have chosen. Advertising through leaflet drops, newspapers, local radio, etc., will need little, if any, equipment, whereas salon displays, demonstrations and shows will require access to specific hairdressing tools and equipment. Always ensure that any tools, equipment, products – and staff – are available not only on the night of the demonstration or show but also during any rehearsals.

Promotional materials and products

Promotional materials include posters, leaflets, tickets, programmes and vouchers. These will all have to be printed, and some will be needed sooner than others, so it is a good idea to make up a production schedule for each item, and to give a member of the team responsibility for ensuring that dates are adhered to.

> To celebrate the opening of our new Hairdressing & Beauty Salon,
> join us for an evening of Creativity and Innovation with
> **PATRICK CAMERON**
> On Tuesday 26th October 2004
> at 6.30pm for 7.00pm
> RSVP Stephanie Henderson 0208 756 0414
> by 7th October
> Hayes Centre, Coldharbour Lane, Hayes,
> Middlesex UB3 3BB
> THIS TICKET ADMITS ONE PERSON

Invitation to a salon promotion

If you are promoting a particular product or range of products, make sure that you have sufficient supplies in stock for retail, and also for use in demonstrations or shows (including rehearsals). Contact product manufacturers to see if they are willing to provide free samples for clients to try, or for use during a demonstration or show.

HEALTH MATTERS
Always take into account health and safety considerations and any other legal requirements when planning your promotional activity. Remember to give a member of the team responsibility for overseeing health and safety.

Demonstrations and shows

Two major factors when deciding on the format of a demonstration or hair show are the type and size of audience you wish to attract.

Demonstrations

Demonstrations are usually aimed at smaller groups. Audiences will fall into two categories: professional and non-professional.

Professional groups

These could be made up of your staff or hairdressers from other salons – either experienced stylists or trainees. For groups of this type, the content of the demonstration would be more technical – perhaps a demonstration of a particular technique or skill.

Remember to take into account the abilities of the group when planning the content of the demonstration.

Non-professional groups

Non-professional audiences can be from specific organisations such as Women's Institutes, Girl Guides or mother-and-toddler groups. The age of the audience needs to be considered when planning this type of event.

These demonstrations would be more informal and could include hair and beauty make-overs, question-and-answer sessions on hair and beauty, one-to-one consultations, and also information on the services your salon offers.

Although the two groups are very different, the methods of preparation and presentation of the demonstration are similar.

Shows

If you choose to present a larger show it is important to reach a good cross-section of the community. One possibility would be to involve a local charity and use the show as a fund-raising event.

The size of the presentation will also influence your choice of venue, the content of the show and the price of entry tickets.

Content

One of the first decisions that must be made is the format and content of the show. A brainstorming session with members of your team is a good way of coming up with ideas.

Some possibilities include:

- Hair and fashion, using mature and young models
- A children's event
- Weddings
- Sports
- Avant-garde
- High fashion
- Historical themes
- Make-over spot.

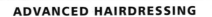

TO DO

Think of some other 'themes' that could be incorporated into your show.

Once you have decided on the content of the show, your next step is to plan the sequence and pace of the delivery. In discussion with members of your team, decide on the sequence of the themes chosen and the length of time each segment should last.

Remember, you are showing your skills to prospective clients. Don't rush the delivery or it will be difficult for the audience to take in what they are seeing. On the other hand, don't let things drag on for too long or the audience may lose interest.

Rehearsals will give a good idea as to how things are progressing and allow adjustments to be made.

Putting a show together

There will be various costs involved in putting a hair show together and these will depend greatly on the size of the presentation planned.

Costs may include:

- Cost of hiring the venue
- Printing of promotional materials
- Publicity – advertisements in local newspapers, etc.
- Accessories – hair ornamentation, hairpieces, jewellery, etc.
- Hair products – shampoos, styling products, etc.
- Sundry items – dry-cleaning, laundry, refreshments, etc.
- Fees for helpers.

One way of reducing costs would be to involve local businesses in the event. For example:

- Local clothes/shoe stores could be asked to loan outfits
- Design students from the local college might help with designing promotional materials; fashion students could design outfits for avant-garde themes
- Bridal shops could lend outfits for a wedding theme
- Record stores may help with music
- Local radio may give free advertising
- Local papers may print an article about the salon and the show
- Inviting local businesses and hair-product manufacturers/retailers to advertise in the programme will help reduce printing costs
- If you don't know any make-up artists, get in touch with local beauty salons or freelance artists.

Example of Cost Estimates for a College Hair Show

Lighting and sound £150

Hair accessories £80

Video production £40

Photography £50

Programmes . . . . Donated by Wella

Security . . . . All staff gave services free

Refreshments £150

Hall hire . . . . Free

Hair sundries (gel, spray, etc.) £20

Flowers £30

Raffle prize . . . . CD player from Wella was bonus offer

Printing costs £20

Choosing the date

The timing of the show may be influenced by several factors:

- Availability of the venue. You may be restricted by available dates so check with the venue before setting a firm date.
- Holidays. Remember to take into account staff, school and public holidays.
- Time of year. If planning a show during the winter months, remember that the weather may affect the size of the audience.

Choosing the venue

Several factors will need to be considered when choosing a suitable venue:

- It must be easily accessible. Are there good public transport and car parking facilities? Facilities and access for the disabled?
- Is the hall big enough for your needs? Remember to find out the maximum audience capacity.
- Does it have the facilities you require? These will include a stage area, adequate seating, a changing area with room for preparation of models, suitable water and power supply and appropriate lighting. Remember to check out the sound system. Is there one you can use, or will you have to supply your own?
- How much will it cost? Are there reduced rates for certain days of the week or times of the year? If possible, check out several places – sports centres, community centres, school halls or hotels – and compare prices before deciding on a venue.
- Are you allowed to use the venue for rehearsals?
- Will the venue be ready for use on the date required (for example, will seating be provided), or are you responsible for setting up?

Publicising the show

There are many ways to publicise the show and it is important that whichever methods you choose will reach a large number of people. Possible ideas include mailshots to homes within the area, or leaflets/fliers delivered with local free papers. A press release or advertisement in the local papers with details of date and time will create interest, as would a spot on a local radio show. Promotional posters displayed throughout the area are also a good idea.

Allocating jobs

Listed below are some of the roles which need to be undertaken by members of your team:

- **Show co-ordinator** – this involves overseeing the whole event and liaising with all those involved in the show.
- **Compere** – needs to be a good communicator and comfortable speaking to a large group of people.
- **Stylists** – must be confident working in front of people, competent and able to choose styles for models that can be easily converted backstage. They also need to be able to work quickly – time is often limited.

- **Juniors** – needed to assist backstage with minor tasks and preparation work. Must be able to take instruction, work with minimum support and use initiative.
- **Make-up artists** – needed to make up models. (Note: If any make-up artists are new to you, make sure you see examples of their work before agreeing to use them. Try approaching local colleges/beauty salons for help.)
- **Dresser** – needed to co-ordinate outfits and accessories.
- **Models** – must be confident and able to perform routines and walk the catwalk without embarrassment.
- **Choreographer** – needed to plan routines, timing of models, etc.
- **Music co-ordinator** – needs to be familiar with music systems and able to suggest suitable music for each theme.
- **IT support co-ordinator** – to help with computer-aided graphics for any back projections.

Problems

As with any activity, problems may arise. Below are some problems which may arise and ways of avoiding them.

POTENTIAL HAZARD	PRECAUTIONS TO REDUCE HEALTH AND SAFETY RISKS
Overload of electricity supply Unchecked electrical equipment	Have supply and equipment checked beforehand by a qualified electrician
Models' accessories may have sharp, pointed ends	Use with care
Spillages caused by using basins not designed for shampooing	Wipe up spillages immediately
Possible allergies to make-up products	Use hypo-allergenic products
Trailing wires and flexes	Use tape or other appropriate means to secure
Work areas becoming untidy	Designate people to continually tidy up
Audience exceeds maximum numbers stated in fire regulations	Restrict numbers allowed to enter
Not knowing where fire exits are situated	Learn location in advance and inform audience at the beginning of the presentation
Not knowing where the fire equipment is situated	Learn location and how to use in advance
Clothing may be made of old fabrics which may not be fire resistant	Avoid proximity to fire sources
Added hair made from inflammable man-made fibres	Avoid proximity to fire sources
Possible allergy to glue used to attach added hair	Conduct skin test before using
Unprofessional removal of added hair causing client discomfort and possible hair and scalp damage	Use only trained staff with the correct equipment to remove added hair

REMEMBER

Salon staff and clients could be used as models. Alternatively, contact model agencies if the budget allows.

TO DO

Using the list of roles, consider the tasks each person would be expected to carry out before and during the show.

TO DO

Think of ways to resolve the problems below, and think of some other problems which may arise and how to solve them:
- *You've run out of promotional materials and products*
- *The venue has been double booked*
- *Jobs not carried out to schedule*
- *Promotional materials not ready on time*
- *Resources, e.g. stock, not available*
- *Models let you down*
- *Staff/models late for rehearsals.*

Evaluation and assessment of the activity

Evaluation and assessment of your promotional activity will help you to gauge its success and learn lessons for future promotions.

Reasons for evaluation and assessment

- **Qualitative** – to gain feedback on the activity. Was the quality of the promotion better than previous promotions? Was it as good as, or worse than, those of your competitors?
- **Quantitative** – to judge the effect on salon training. Were the resources – tools, equipment, products and promotional materials – adequate?

There are many methods of evaluation. Some examples are given below:

- Feedback/discussion sessions with other members of the team
- Informal talks with clients – these will give a general overview of how people felt about the promotion
- Keeping a record of new clients visiting the salon
- Monitoring sales of services or products promoted to see if there is an increase in demand
- Questionnaires – these give more structured feedback and can be designed for both staff and clients to complete.

Managers need to keep records of evaluations and assessments to be able to justify and improve future promotions.

Whatever form of evaluation you choose, the following topics should be included:

- Did the activity achieve its aims and objectives? (Was it valid?)
- Costs involved: how was money spent? Could it have been better spent elsewhere?
- What do you think worked well? (Were the techniques current?)
- Are there any areas that could be improved? (Was it authentic?)
- Content: would you use the same format again?
- Was there anything that should be added, or left out, next time? (Was it sufficient?)

If a hair show/demonstration:

- Was the pace too fast/slow/OK?
- Method of delivery: was it clear and concise? Did the audience understand what was going on?

On page 238 you will find an example of an evaluation questionnaire.

Reviewing the evaluation questionnaire

The completed evaluation questionnaire sheets need to be compiled by adding up the amounts of 'yes' and 'no' responses to give percentages. For example:

Q1	Did you enjoy the show?

TO DO

Once you have chosen your promotional activity, design an evaluation questionnaire which could be given to clients and/or staff to complete.

If 80 people attended and 75 answered 'yes' and 5 answered 'no' then 94% enjoyed the show but 6% did not.

Working out percentages

A percentage is another way of writing a fraction. Per cent means 'out of 100'.

Simply, 10% is one-tenth (1/10) of 100; 20% is two-tenths (2/10) of 100. Unfortunately not all percentages are as simple as this. To express a number as a percentage of another number you have to convert the figures into fractions. For example, to find a percentage for 36 out of 50, convert this to the fraction 36/50. Because a percentage is out of 100 we need to change the fraction to 100ths. If we multiply 50 by two we get 100; so then we must also multiply 36 by two. This gives 72/100 = 72%.

Likewise, to write 14 out of 20 as a percentage, change the 20 to 100 by multiplying by 5. Then multiply 14 by 5 = 70%.

This can also be done using a calculator. For 36 out of 50, enter 36 divided by 50 then multiply by 100. For 14 out of 20, enter 14 divided by 20 then multiply by 100.

Audience comments should also be clearly and logically listed, e.g. it needs to be stated only once that five people said that the commentary could have been a little louder.

Both positive and negative feedback of a general nature can be given:

- Through general discussion – informally in the staff restroom during breaks or formally during staff meetings.

- In a written form – through staff appraisals (see Chapter 10), where confidentiality is needed (especially if feedback is negative). Always make your feedback constructive and put the other person at ease – most people realise when they have made a mistake and are only too anxious to improve any future performances. Allow the staff to provide their own suggestions on how they could improve, and list the ideas as part of their future goals.

- By using IT skills to collate, analyse and summarise in a clear and concise way using text, spreadsheets, graphs or pie/bar charts.

TEST YOUR KNOWLEDGE

1 List the main reasons for promoting a salon.

2 List the ways of promoting a salon.

3 How do you decide on what type of promotional activity to use?

4 Describe the difference between someone who works within the line manager's responsibility and someone who has a functional responsibility, and the implications these differences may have for planning the work.

5 Why is it important to plan and prepare a promotional activity?

6 Why is it important to involve staff/colleagues?

7 How would you suit staff to specific tasks?

8 List the ways of publicising your promotion.

9 Why is it a good idea to evaluate promotions and shows?

10 How can you evaluate the success of your promotion to ensure that it is a fair and objective assessment?

11 How could both negative and positive feedback be given and why is it important?

12 Which type of feedback should always be confidential and why?

13 How does the evaluation of your promotion apply to you (the manager)?

Hair and Beauty Show Evaluation

Please spare two minutes to complete this questionnaire to let us know what you thought about the show.
Please tick the Yes or No boxes:

		Yes	No
1	Did you enjoy the show?	☐	☐
2	Could you see everything clearly?	☐	☐
3	Could you hear everything that was said?	☐	☐
4	Did you find it easy to purchase the tickets?	☐	☐
5	Was the Level 2 (the full-time students') work up to the standard you expected?	☐	☐
6	Was the Level 3 (mature students') work up to the standard you expected?	☐	☐
7	Did you find the college map helpful?	☐	☐
8	Was the price of the ticket good value for money?	☐	☐
9	Were the refreshments sufficient?	☐	☐
10	If we put on another show next year, will you come?	☐	☐

Please feel free to add any other comments below:

_____

_____

_____

Name _____

Signature _____ Date _____

Index